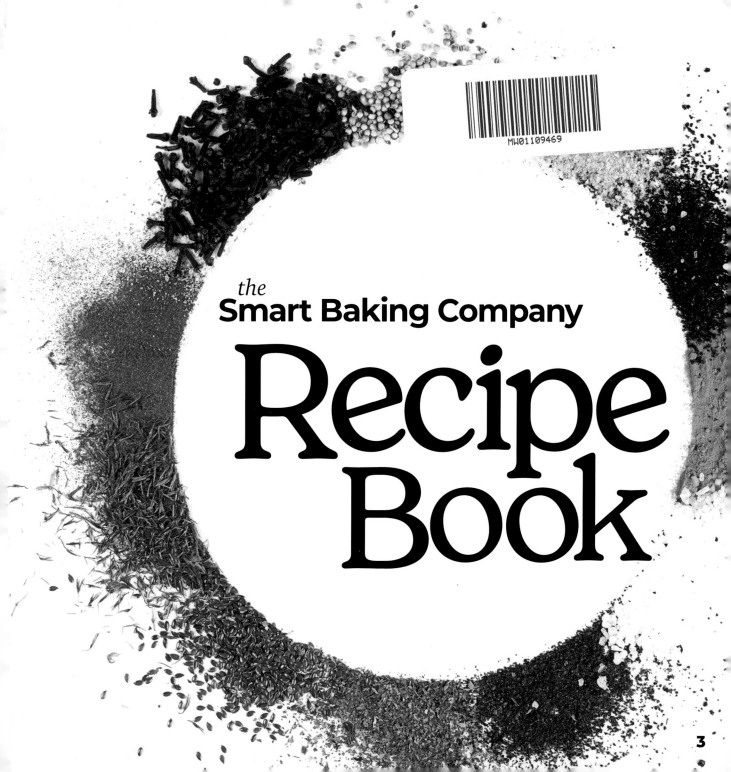

the
Smart Baking Company

Recipe Book

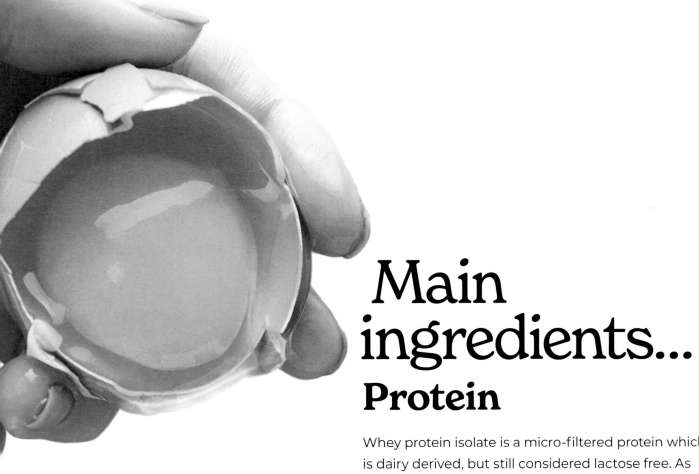

Main ingredients...
Protein

Whey protein isolate is a micro-filtered protein which is dairy derived, but still considered lactose free. As published in the Journal of Sports Science & Medicine and the NIH, it is a complete, high-quality protein, containing all of the essential amino acids. In addition, it is very digestible, absorbed by the gut quickly compared to other types of protein.

Eggs are another source of protein in our products. Unlike most cereals and yogurt, eggs only contain one ingredient – "eggs." No sugar or carbs, just high quality protein. And protein in our meals ensures that we truly feel satiated.

Pure Water

A well hydrated body is 70% water. Smartcakes® and Smartbuns® also have water as a key ingredient and not water laden with added chemicals. We use nano filtering systems created by actual rocket scientists to ensure our water is pure. Better water starts the process for better food. Smart Baking Company partnered with Argonide to use the best water possible. Their Cool Blue® water purifier incorporates three layers of technology to ensure the best tasting and purest water we can use to add to the quality and taste of our products and the nutritional value to you.

Flax Meal

Flax Meal is also a key ingredient in our products and contains Omega-3 essential fatty acids which are according to National Institute of Health (NIH) published studies, the "good" fats that have been shown to have heart-healthy effects. It is also rich in fiber as well as lignans, which have antioxidant qualities. Flaxseed contains 75 to 800 times more lignans than other plant foods.

Olive Oil

Olive Oil is another ingredient that serves up good health. According to the Mayo Clinic, monounsaturated fatty acids (MUFAs), the main type of fat found in olive oil, is considered a healthy dietary fat and may help lower your risk of heart disease by improving related risk factors. MUFAs have been found to lower total cholesterol and low-density lipoprotein (LDL) cholesterol levels. In addition, some research shows that MUFAs may benefit insulin levels and blood sugar control, which can be helpful if you have or are at risk of type 2 diabetes. According to statistics at the NIH as well as recent studies by the Center for Disease Control and Prevention, approximately one in three adult Americans has diabetes or is pre-diabetic.

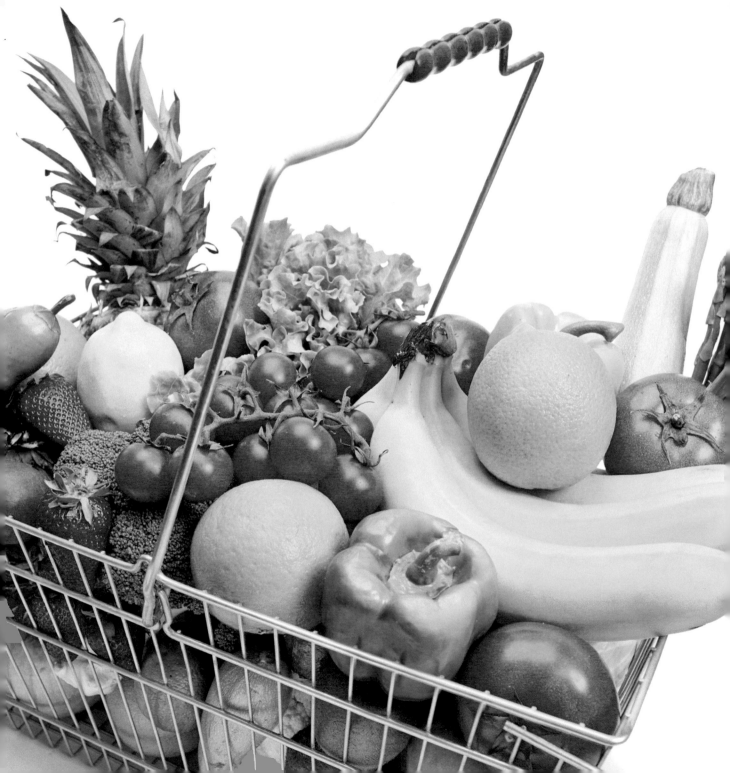

Special ingredients...

Using our Smartbuns® as a base for a burger or as an ingredient in your next meal, saves you time, money and adds a healthy kick to many favorite comfort foods. Now you can be comforted in good health.

How does it save you money? **Let's go shopping.**

If the benefits of a Smartbun® were replicated in a shopping cart, with 10 grams of high-quality protein per bun, you would need:

- 3 ounces of pure, non-GMO protein preferably one high in Omega 3 fats.

- Enough mixed vegetables to get 12 grams of insoluble fiber

- 1/2 of a banana for Potassium

Do all of this without exceeding the 63 good for you calories found in our Smartbuns®

What did we leave out of the cart?
We left out Sugar, Starch, and Glutens.

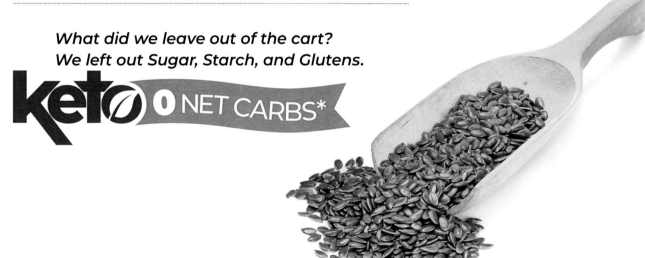

keto 0 NET CARBS*

7

Our whole bakery...

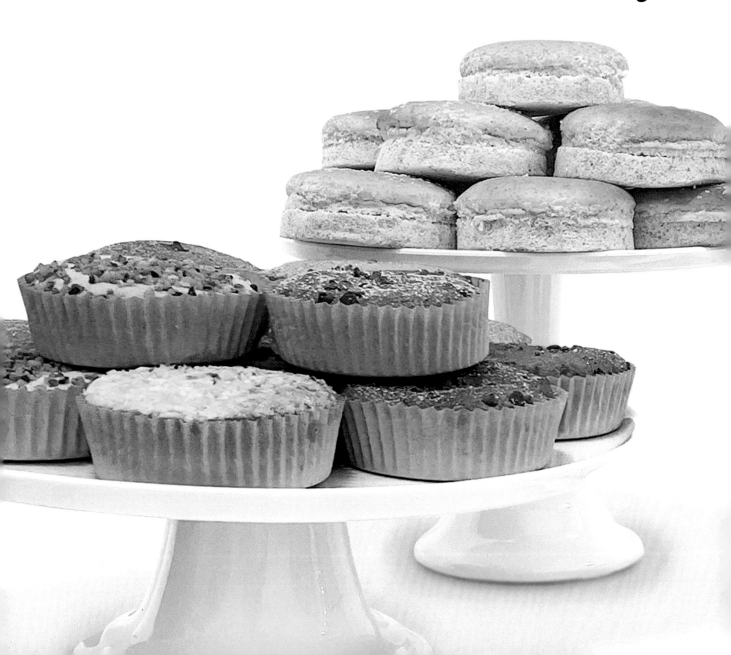

is your foundation.

Just as the Smartbuns® are perfect when toasted and dipped in some garlic infused olive oil as a snack, our Smartmuf'ns® and Smartcakes® replace several ingredients and turn decadent desserts into delicious but actually good for you desserts.

When you taste your first forkful of our Autumn Trifle, you will wonder why you ever wasted time on unhealthy, sugar laden desserts when this one is so delicious, stunning to see and amazingly healthy to eat.

Smartmuf'ns® range from 94 to 113 calories of all good for you ingredients and range from 10-13 grams of insoluble fiber and 8-10 grams of high quality protein respectively.

Smartcakes® are an amazing 38 calories each and provide in those few calories 5 grams of insoluble fiber and 4 grams of high quality protein.

Pick your favorite flavors and recipes or enjoy these Smartmuf'ns® and Smartcakes® on their own. ***Always gluten, starch and sugar free. Always full of good proteins and insoluble fiber. Every meal or snack is another chance to choose taste and health.***

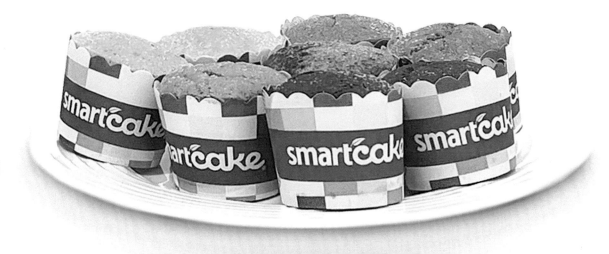

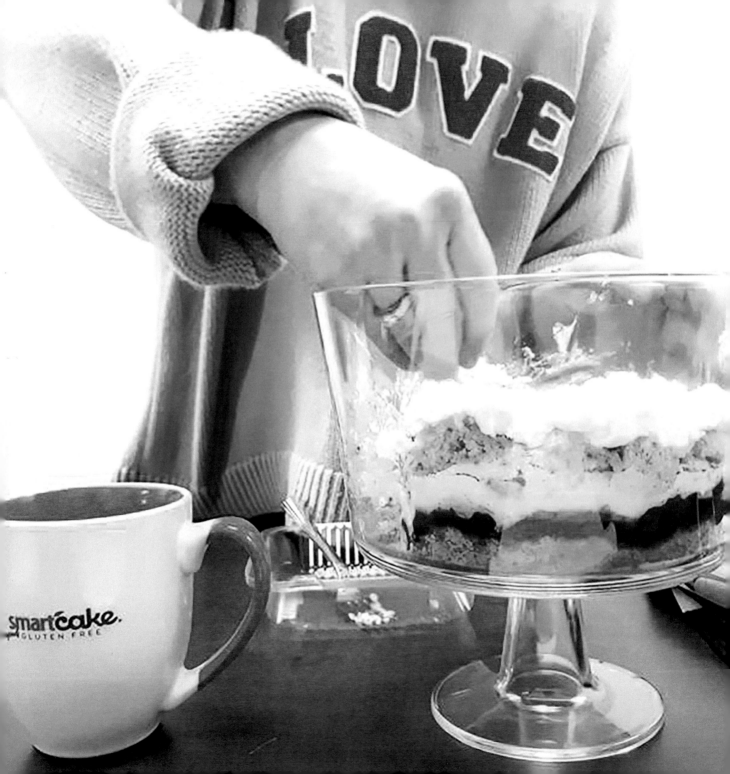

Table of Contents

Breakfast & Snacks

Sandwiches & Burgers

Main & Side Dishes

Desserts

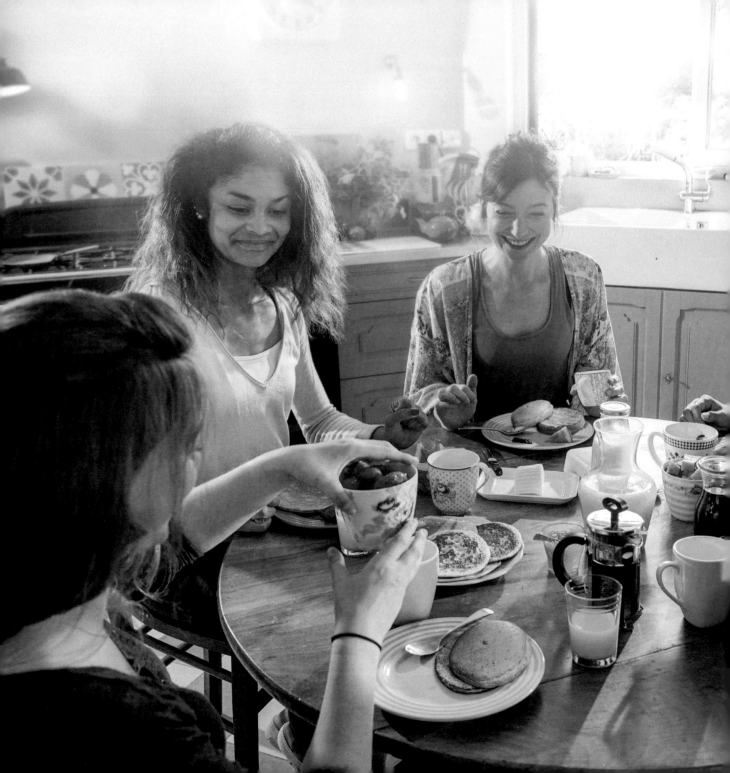

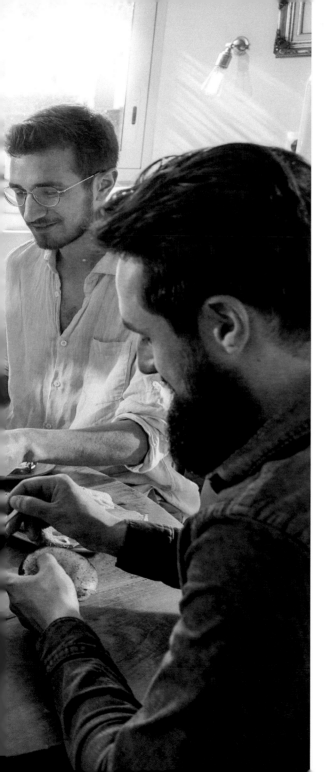

Breakfast
& Snacks

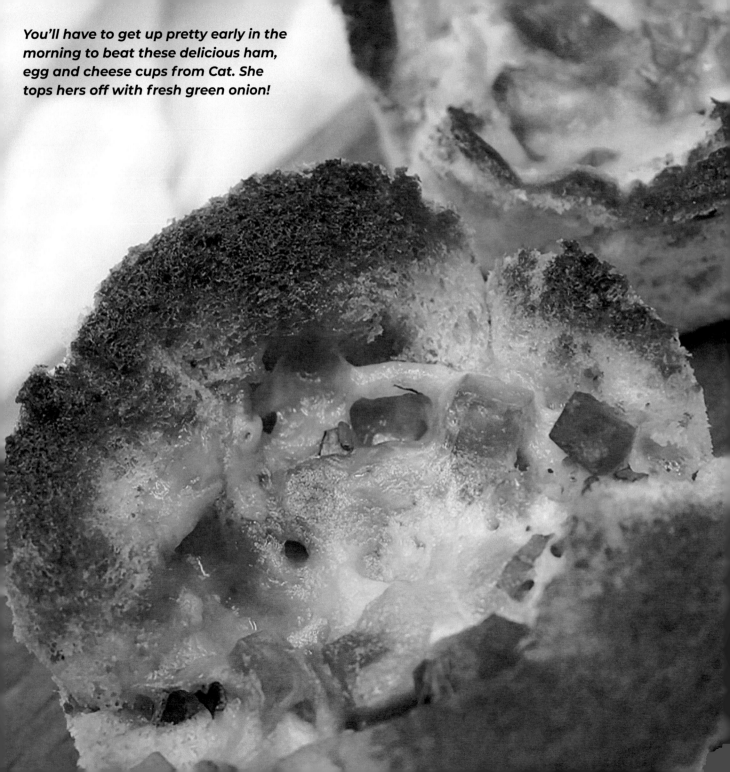

You'll have to get up pretty early in the morning to beat these delicious ham, egg and cheese cups from Cat. She tops hers off with fresh green onion!

Cat's Breakfast Egg Cups

Ingredients:

1 whole egg
2 tbsp diced ham
1 tbsp shredded cheddar cheese
1 tbsp butter

1 plain Smartbun® (makes 2)
Salt & pepper (to taste)
Optional toppings: green onion

Preparation:

1. Preheat oven (or toaster oven) to 350°F.

2. Grease two 1-cup ramekins with cooking spray and set aside.

3. Heat a Plain Smartbun® in the microwave for 15 seconds or until warm.

4. Using a tablespoon, portion 1/2 tbsp pieces of Smartbun® and press firmly into the baking ramekin, forming a well in the center.

5. In a separate bowl, whisk together the egg, cheese, and ham.

6. Pour half of the mixture into each "well" and place in the oven for approximately 15-20 minutes or until the egg has set.

7. Eat directly out of the ramekin or allow the "muffin" to cool slightly and enjoy!

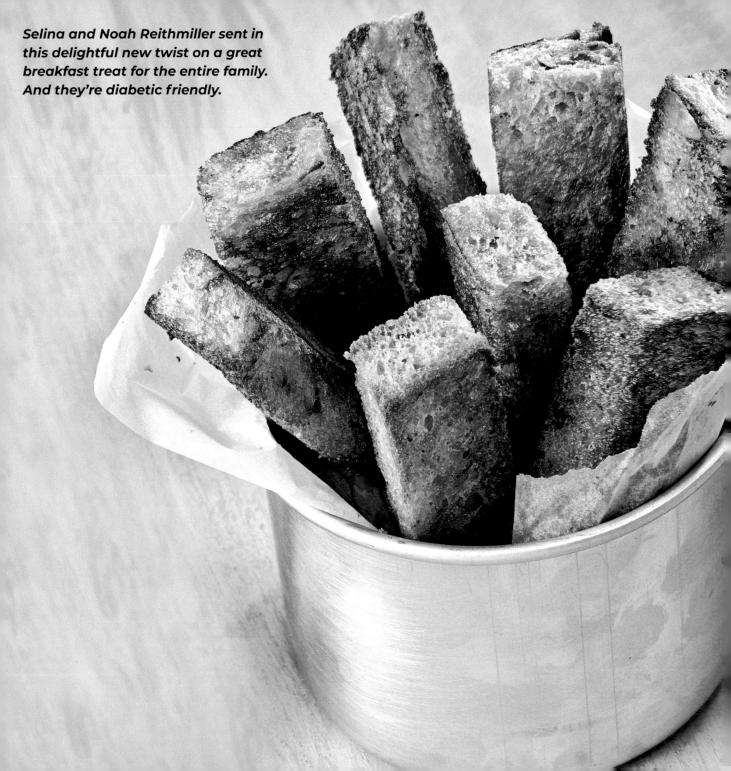

Selina and Noah Reithmiller sent in this delightful new twist on a great breakfast treat for the entire family. And they're diabetic friendly.

Noah's French Toast Sticks

Ingredients:

2 whole eggs - scrambled
1 cup of unsweetened dairy-free milk
A pinch of cinnamon spice
2 tbsp of butter or margarine
2 plain Smartbuns®

Preparation:

1. Add milk and eggs in a large mixing bowl and scramble using a fork or whisk.

2. Take the Plain Smartbuns® out of their wrappers and cut into mini-strips for the French toast sticks.

3. Soak the Smartbun® pieces in the egg and milk mix, then sprinkle with cinnamon.

4. Add butter to skillet and cook the mini-strips on medium heat for approximately 2-3 minutes on each side, or until crispy and golden brown.

5. For an added treat serve with fresh fruit!

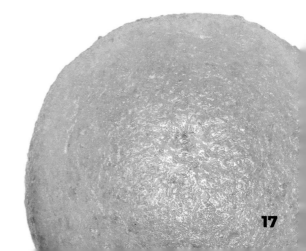

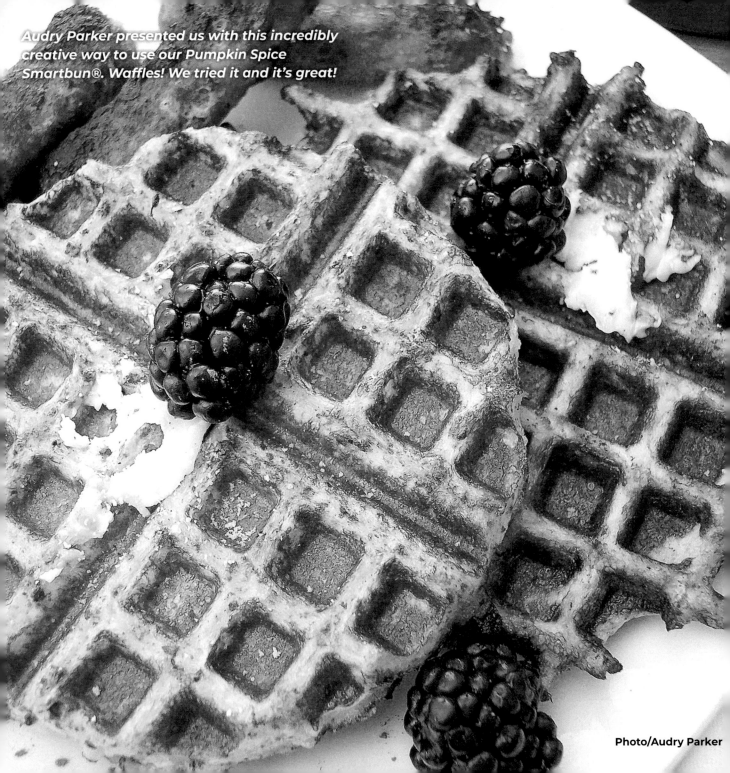

Audry Parker presented us with this incredibly creative way to use our Pumpkin Spice Smartbun®. Waffles! We tried it and it's great!

Photo/Audry Parker

Audrey's Pumpkin Waffles

Ingredients:

1 whole egg
1/4 cup dairy-free milk
1 tsp granulated sweetener
1/2 tsp pumpkin spice extract

1/8 tsp cinnamon
1/8 tsp ground cloves
1/8 tsp butter
1 plain Smartbun® - toasted

Preparation:

1. Toast the Smartbun® to keep it's consistency through the next steps.

2. Grease and heat your waffle iron per manufacturer's directions.

3. Whisk together egg, milk, sweetener, extract and spices in a small bowl.

4. Dip each slice of Smartbun® on both sides into the mixture. Let the bread sit for approximately

5. 15-30 seconds, making sure it is completely covered.

6. Cook Smartbuns® in the preheated waffle iron for approximately 2-3 minutes or until golden brown.

7. Remove and serve immediately with your choice of toppings such as butter, whipped cream, low carb confectioners' sugar, sugar-free syrup, low carb berries, or ice cream. Or experiment with your own fun toppings!

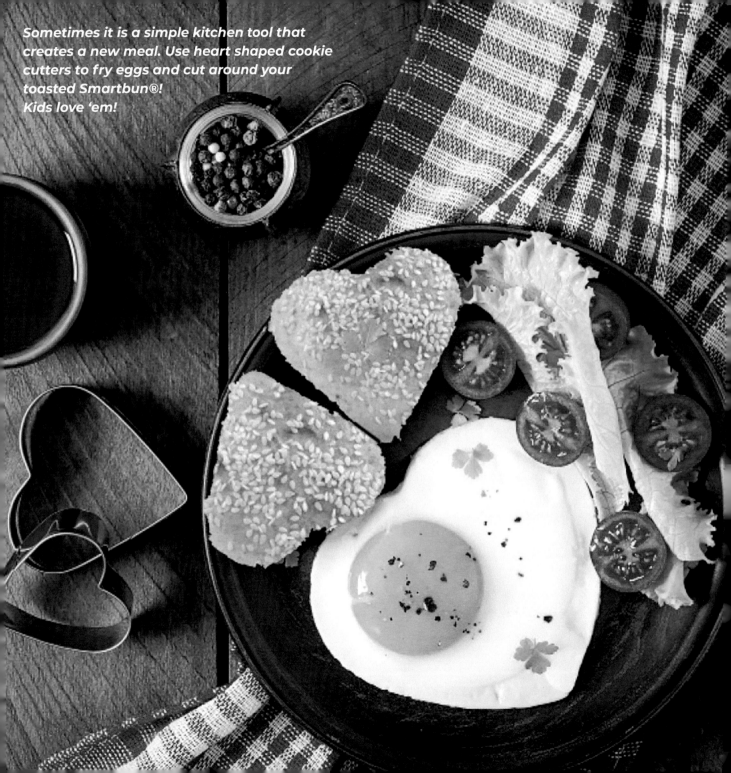

Sometimes it is a simple kitchen tool that creates a new meal. Use heart shaped cookie cutters to fry eggs and cut around your toasted Smartbun®!
Kids love 'em!

Cookie Cutter Breakfast

Ingredients:

1 SmartBun®
2 eggs
Preferred spices and sides

Preparation:

1. Cook an egg any way you like it using a heart shaped cookie cuter! Or be adventurous and use any shape cookie cutter you like! We made our eggs over easy.

2. Use another cookie cutter to cut around your toasted Smartbun® for a health and loving start to the day.

3. Enjoy! Anyone would love this fun and creative take on a healthy breakfast but kids love them especially!

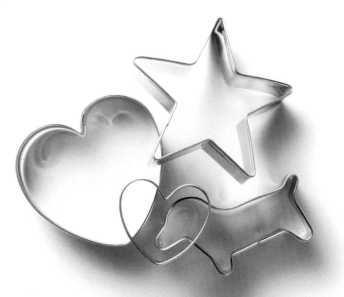

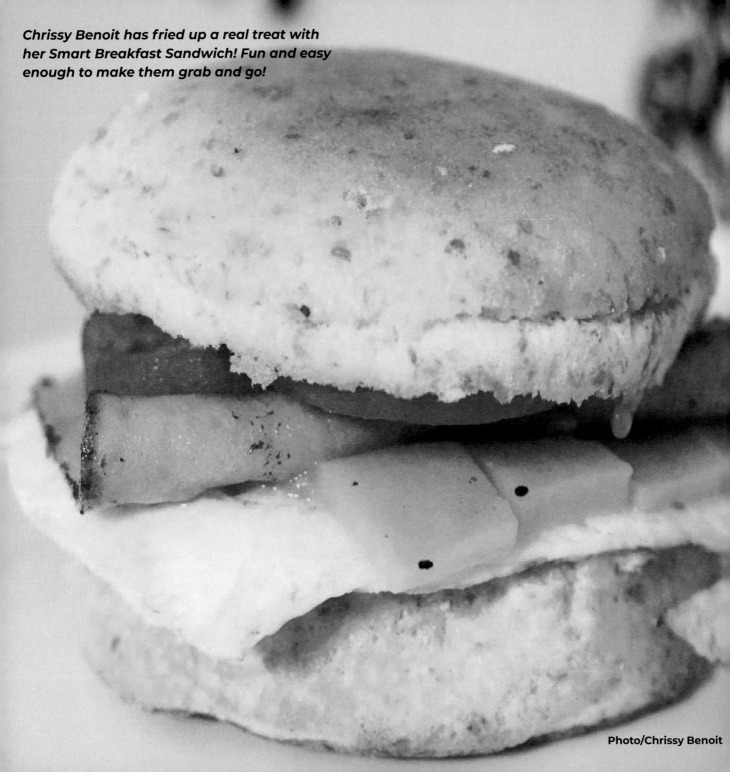

Chrissy Benoit has fried up a real treat with her Smart Breakfast Sandwich! Fun and easy enough to make them grab and go!

Photo/Chrissy Benoit

Chrissy's Smart Breakfast

Ingredients:

1 Smartbun®
1 egg
2 deli meat slices
2 tomato slices

1 cheese slice
Salt and pepper to taste
2-3 Tbsp mayo

Preparation:

1. Fry an egg in a frying pan with butter, coconut oil or palm oil.

2. Break yolk and fry until evenly cooked (unless you like it runny of course).

3. Spread Mayo on your Smartbun® (toast if you'd like), top with egg, 2 thin slices of tomato, deli meat (optional), cheese and season to taste with salt and pepper.

4. Serve and enjoy--so quick, so easy!

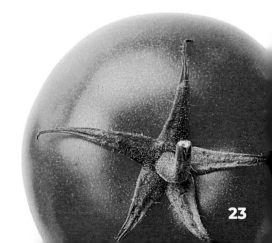

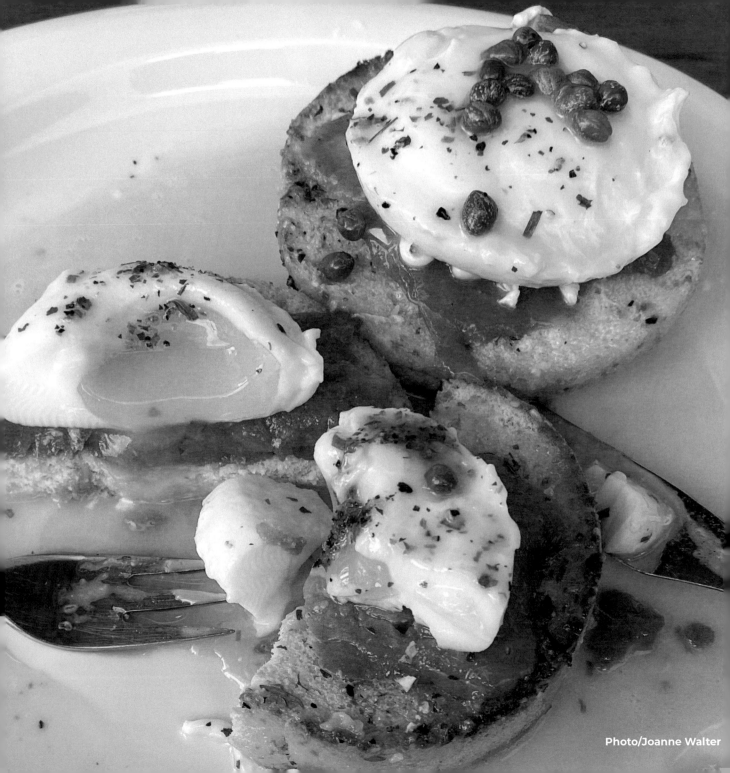

Keto Eggs Benedict with Smoked Salmon

Ingredients:

4 eggs
2 tbsp white balsamic vinegar
2 Plain Smartbuns®, halved

For the hollandaise sauce:
2 tsp lemon juice
2 tsp white balsamic vinegar
3 egg yolks
125g grass-fed, unsalted butter, diced

Grass-fed, unsalted butter as desired
8 slices smoked salmon
chopped chives or capers, to serve

Prep: 15 mins
Cook: 20 mins

Preparation:

1. First make the hollandaise sauce. Combine lemon juice, vinegar, and egg yolks in a small bowl and whisk until light and frothy. Place the bowl over a pan of simmering water and whisk until mixture thickens. Gradually add butter, whisking constantly until it thickens. Season and keep warm.

2. To poach the eggs, bring a large pan of water to the boil and add the vinegar. Lower the heat so that the water is simmering gently. Stir the water so you have a slight whirlpool, then slide in the eggs one by one. Cook each for about 4 mins, then remove with a slotted spoon.

3. Lightly toast and butter the Smartbuns®, then put a couple of slices of salmon on each half. Top each with an egg, spoon over some hollandaise and garnish with chopped chives or capers.

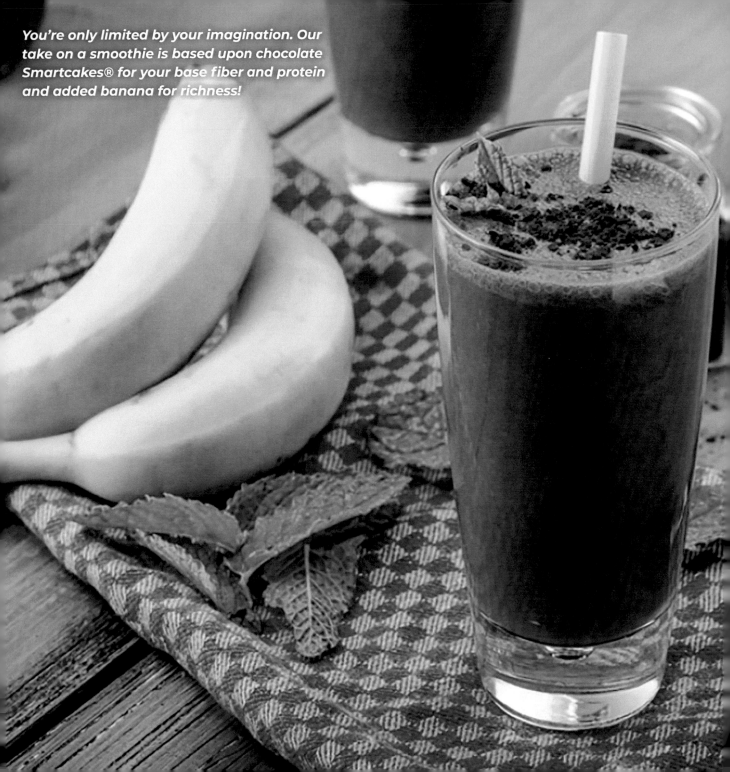

You're only limited by your imagination. Our take on a smoothie is based upon chocolate Smartcakes® for your base fiber and protein and added banana for richness!

Banana Choco-Mint Smoothie

Ingredients:

1 banana
2 chocolate Smartcakes®
1/2 cup unsweetened almond milk

Preparation:

Simply add the ingredients in a high-speed blender and process, pour and enjoy.

Or use the following ingredients for a tropical twist.
1 Banana, 2 Coconut Smartcakes®, 1/2 Cup Unsweetened almond Milk, 1/2 Cup Mango chunks, About 1 Cup, Ice cubes, A few Mint leaves

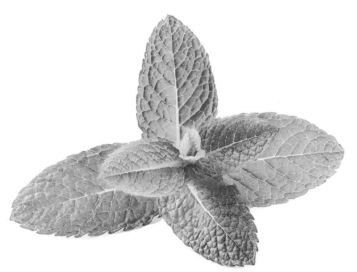

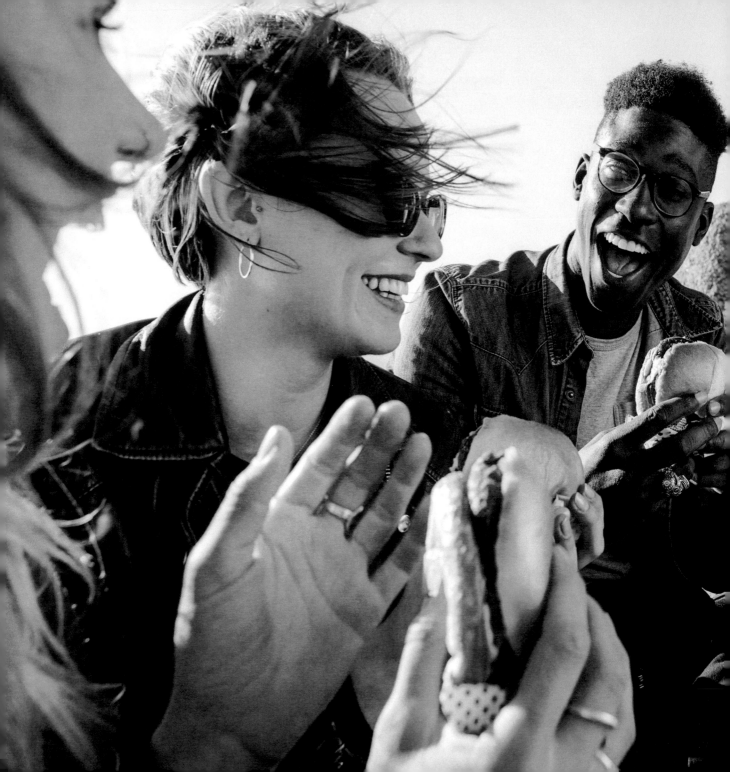

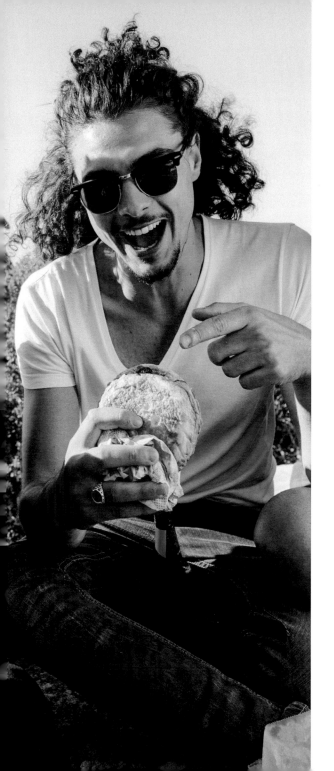

Sandwiches & Burgers

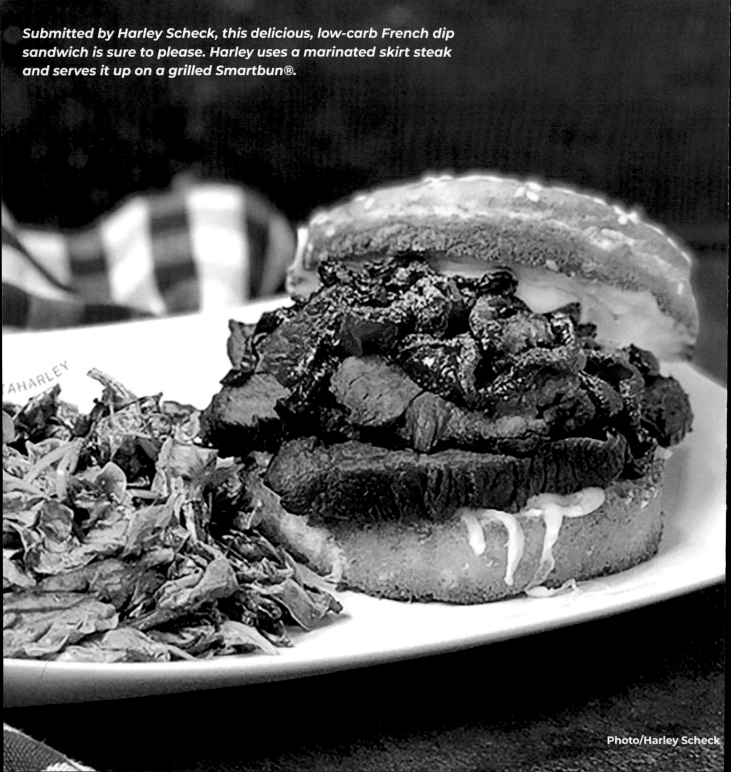

Submitted by Harley Scheck, this delicious, low-carb French dip sandwich is sure to please. Harley uses a marinated skirt steak and serves it up on a grilled Smartbun®.

Photo/Harley Scheck

Harley's French Dip

Ingredients:

4 oz skirt steak
2 large cloves of garlic - minced
1/2 cup onions - sliced
1/4 cup mozzarella - shredded
1/4 cup beef broth

2 tsp butter
2 tsp Worcestershire sauce
2 tsp grated Parmesan cheese
1 tsp your preferred browning sauce
A pinch of salt & pepper

Preparation:

1. Season steak with salt and pepper, half of the minced or grated garlic, 1 tsp of Worcestershire and browning sauce. Marinate 30 minutes.

2. Broil meat to desired internal temperature. Caramelize onions - set aside.

3. Toast Smartbun® with butter, minced garlic and Parmesan cheese 3-5 min.

4. Remove buns from oven and top each inside half with mozzarella cheese. Return to oven to melt cheese.

5. Prepare the au jus in a pan with the sliced onions, beef broth, steak drippings and Worcestershire sauce. Bring to boil, reduce heat and simmer for 2-3 minutes.

6. Slice the steak and place on garlic bread with the onions. Serve with the au jus on the side and enjoy!

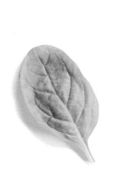
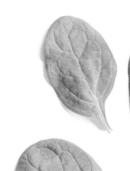
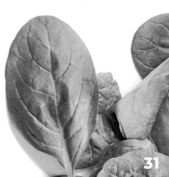

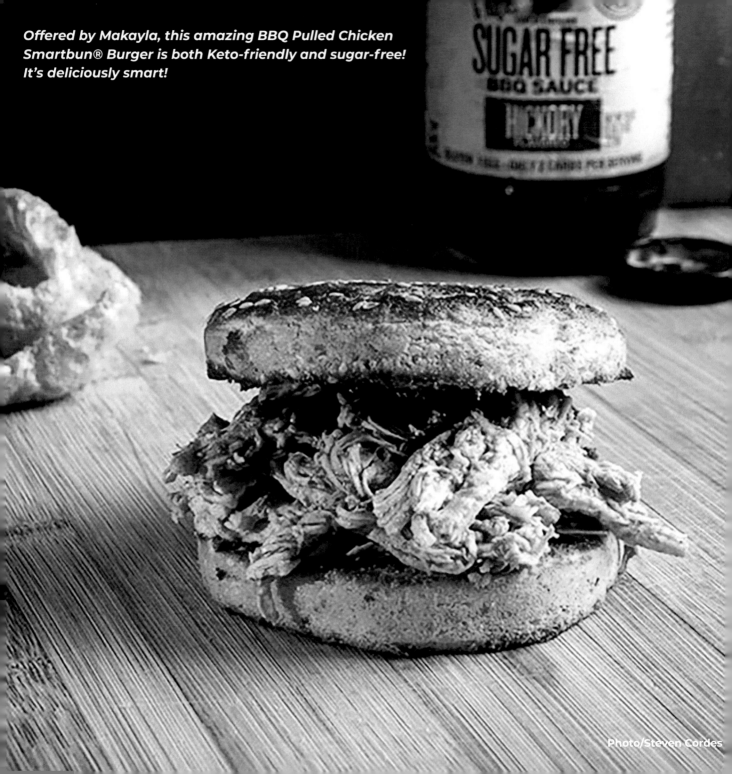

Offered by Makayla, this amazing BBQ Pulled Chicken Smartbun® Burger is both Keto-friendly and sugar-free! It's deliciously smart!

Photo/Steven Cordes

Makayla's Pulled Chicken

Ingredients:

4 Smartbuns®
2.5 lbs raw chicken breasts
8 tbsp sugar-free BBQ sauce
A pinch of salt & pepper

A pinch of onion & garlic powder
1 cup water
1 tbsp of butter
2 oz. mustard

Preparation:

1. Place the chicken in a slow cooker with water and season to taste.
   (salt, pepper, onion, garlic)

2. Add in 4 tbsp of sugar-free BBQ sauce to the instant pot or slow cooker
   and lightly stir until mixed.

3. Cook on manual setting for approximately 20 minutes. (adjust time for a slow cooker)

4. After cooking for 20 minutes, take the chicken out. Place the cooked chicken in a large
   mixing bowl and shred with 2 forks.

5. Add in 4 tbsp more of sugar-free BBQ sauce and mix it in the shredded chicken.

6. Lightly toast the Smartbun® with 1 tbsp of butter or margarine in a skillet on low to
   medium setting, until a crisp golden brown.

7. Layer the shredded BBQ chicken on top of the toasted Smartbuns® and enjoy!

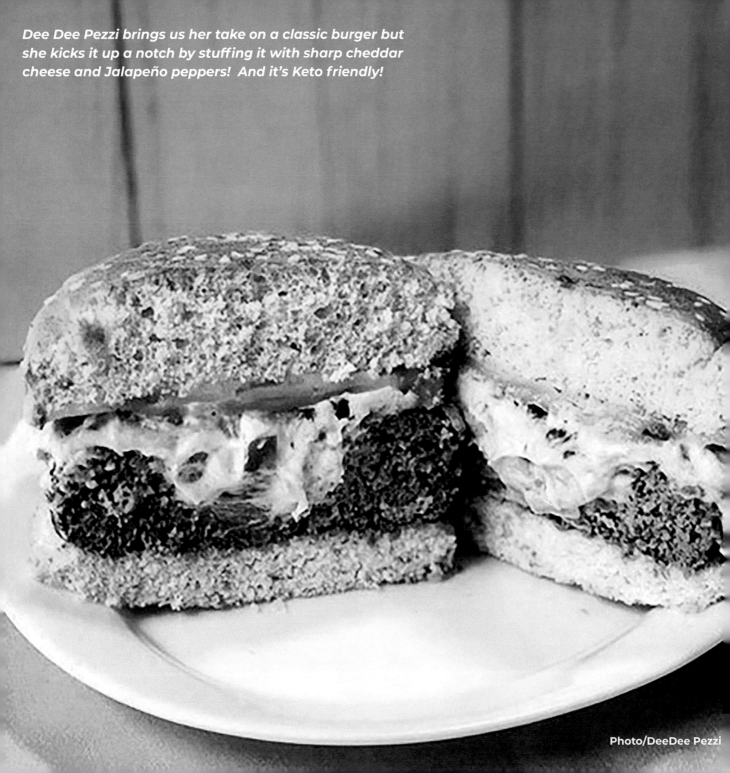

Dee Dee Pezzi brings us her take on a classic burger but she kicks it up a notch by stuffing it with sharp cheddar cheese and Jalapeño peppers! And it's Keto friendly!

Photo/DeeDee Pezzi

Dee Dee's Pepper Poppers

Ingredients:

2 lbs raw ground Beef
Pinch of Salt & Pepper
Pinch of Onion & Garlic powder
8 oz Cream Cheese

1/2 cup shredded sharp cheddar cheese
2 whole Jalapeños (diced)
1/4 cup (about 8 slices) fresh bacon bits
4 Sesame Smartbuns®

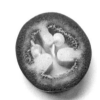

Preparation:

For the stuffing mixture:

1. Cook bacon - dice into bits and set aside.

2. Chop and dice the jalapenos. Set aside.

3. In a large mixing bowl, combine the cream cheese, shredded cheddar cheese, diced bacon and jalapenos.

4. Set completed stuffing mixture aside.

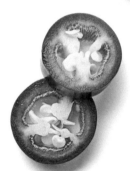

For the burger patties:

1. Season uncooked ground beef to preference.

2. Divide the beef and shape into eight pattys.

3. Spoon the stuffing mixture on to four of the eight patties.

4. Place the remaining four patties on top of the patties that are topped with the stuffing mixture.

5. Using a fork, gently press the edges of the stuffed patties down to seal in the stuffing mixture.

6. Cook the patties to an internal temperature of 165°F.

7. Toast the Smartbuns® with 1 tbsp of butter until a crisp golden brown.

8. Enjoy!

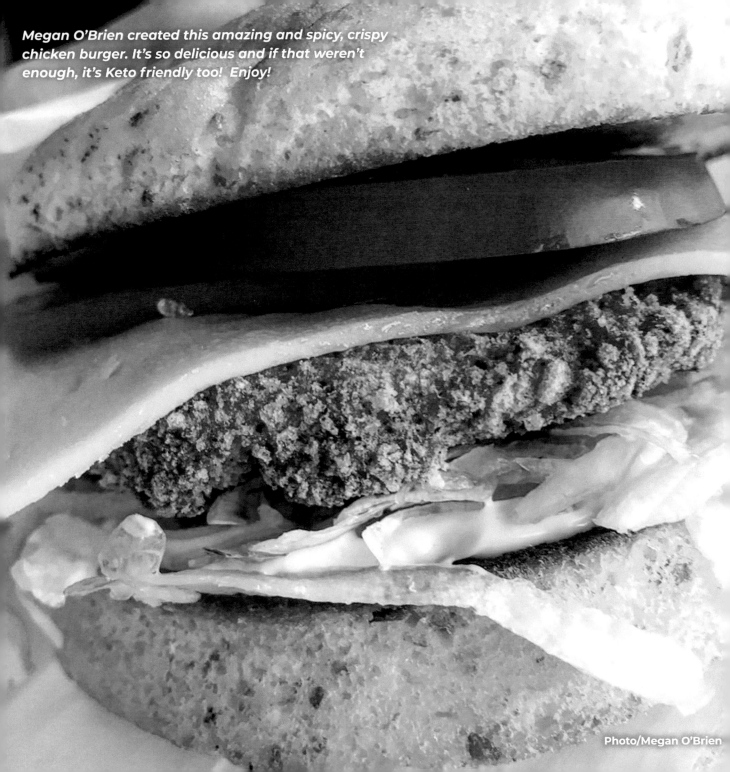

Megan O'Brien created this amazing and spicy, crispy chicken burger. It's so delicious and if that weren't enough, it's Keto friendly too! Enjoy!

Photo/Megan O'Brien

Megan's Crispy Chicken

Ingredients:

1lb of raw ground chicken
1 whole egg
2 tbsp of fresh chives
4 oz gluten-free bread crumb

A pinch of Cajun seasoning
Salt and pepper to taste
6 Smartbuns®

Preparation:

1. Dice the chives.

2. Then mix together the raw ground chicken, egg, salt and pepper.

3. Form six 2.5 oz patties and set in the freezer for approximately 30 minutes.

4. While waiting for the patties to harden, mix the gluten-free bread crumbs with Cajun seasoning.

5. Coat the patties in the crumb mixture, making sure to get all sides thoroughly covered.

6. Air fry at 370 degrees Fahrenheit for approximately 10 minutes on each side to an internal temperature of 165°F. *or* cook on a stove top skillet on medium-high for approximately 10 minutes on each side to an internal temperature of 165°F.

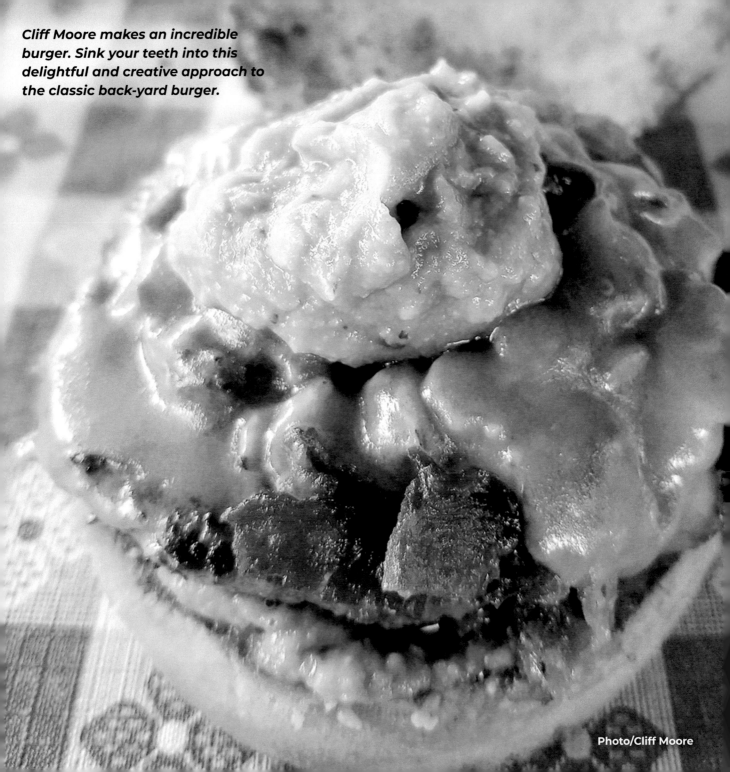

Cliff Moore makes an incredible burger. Sink your teeth into this delightful and creative approach to the classic back-yard burger.

Photo/Cliff Moore

Cliff's Ultimate Keto Burger

Ingredients:

4oz burger patty or ground beef
4 strips bacon
1 whole avocado mashed
1 slice of cheddar cheese

1 oz melted butter
1 sesame Smartbun®
 —(makes one burger)

Preparation:

1. Brush melted butter onto the Smartbun® and grill in a skillet on medium
heat for 1-2 until golden brown.

2. Cook bacon strips in a skillet on medium-high heat for approximately 2 minutes.
Using tongs, flip the bacon and cook for another 2 minutes.

3. Place the cooked bacon on a plate covered with a paper towel to drain.

4. Next either grill or cook the patties on a stove top in a skillet. If using a skillet cook in the
bacon fat for approximately 10 minutes on each side or until
the internal temperature reaches 165°F.

5. Dice bacon and place on top of the burger. Cover with cheese and let it melt over the bacon.

6. Remove from heat and let cool for 2-5 minutes.

7. Place 1/2 the mashed avocado on the bottom of the Smartbun®.

8. Place the burger on top of the avocado, then cheese and the remaining avocado.

9. Layer the Smartbun® over the avocado and enjoy!

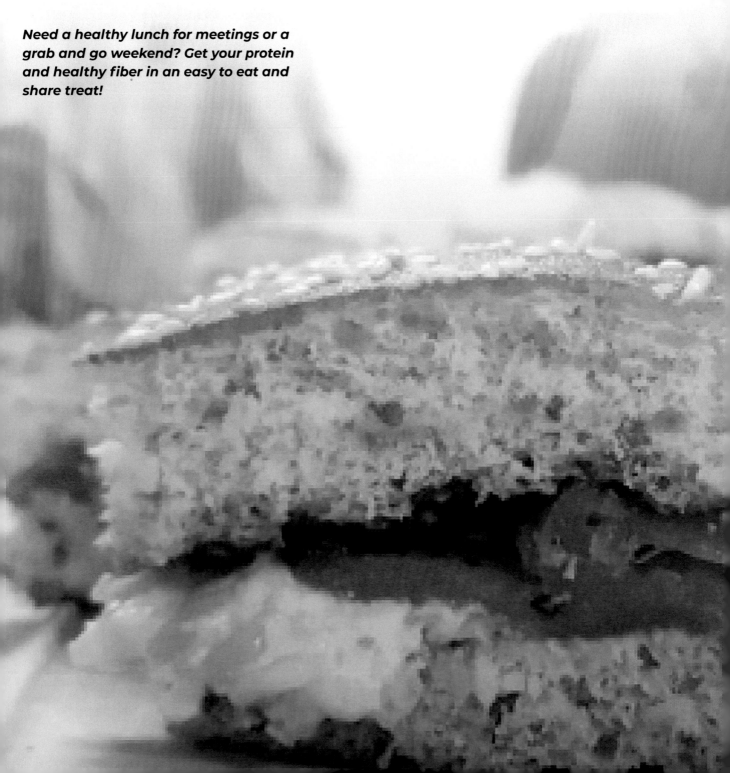

Need a healthy lunch for meetings or a grab and go weekend? Get your protein and healthy fiber in an easy to eat and share treat!

Simply Smart Sandwich

Ingredients:

1 sesame Smartbun®
2 slices smoked salmon
1 slice swiss cheese

2 tbsp pesto sauce
Pinch fresh cilantro
2 tbsp cream cheese

Preparation:

1. Toast a plain or sesame Smartbun®.

2. Add pesto, tomatoes and cheese or Cilantro.

3. Add cream cheese and salmon.

4. Enjoy!

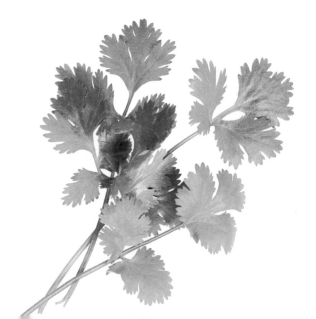

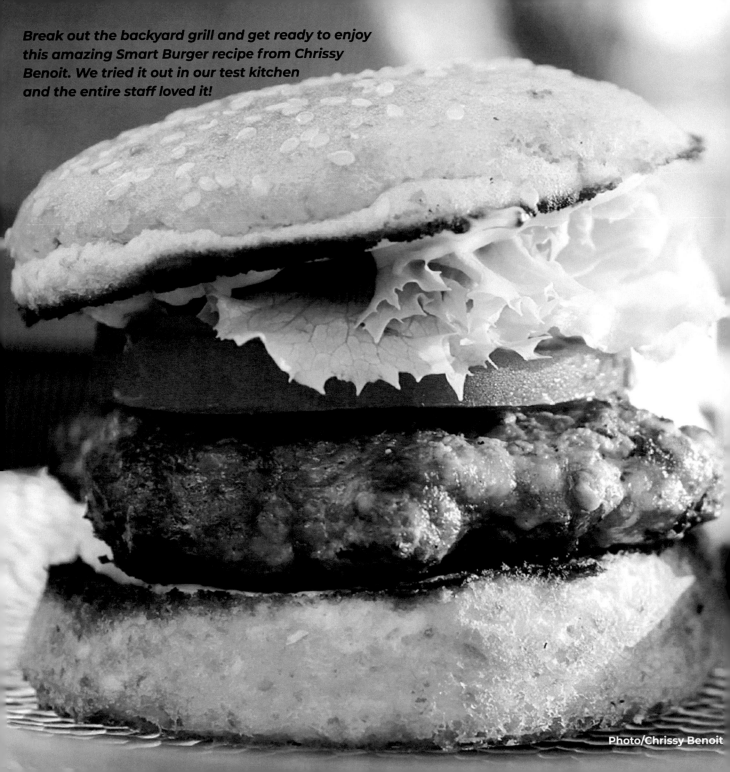

Break out the backyard grill and get ready to enjoy this amazing Smart Burger recipe from Chrissy Benoit. We tried it out in our test kitchen and the entire staff loved it!

Photo/Chrissy Benoit

Chrissy's Smart Burger

Ingredients:

2 lb hamburger meat
1 egg
1 tbsp Onion powder
2 Wasa crackers (crumbled)
2 tsp garlic powder

Salt and pepper to taste
1 cup sharp cheddar cheese (grated)
2 cups chives or green onions
1 Smartbun®

Preparation:

1. In a large bowl, combine all ingredients to thawed hamburger meat.

2. Mix well.

3. Form your patties to the size you'd like.

4. Grill to your preference.

5. Briefly place the Smartbun® on the grill for a quick toast.

6. Add toppings of choice and enjoy!

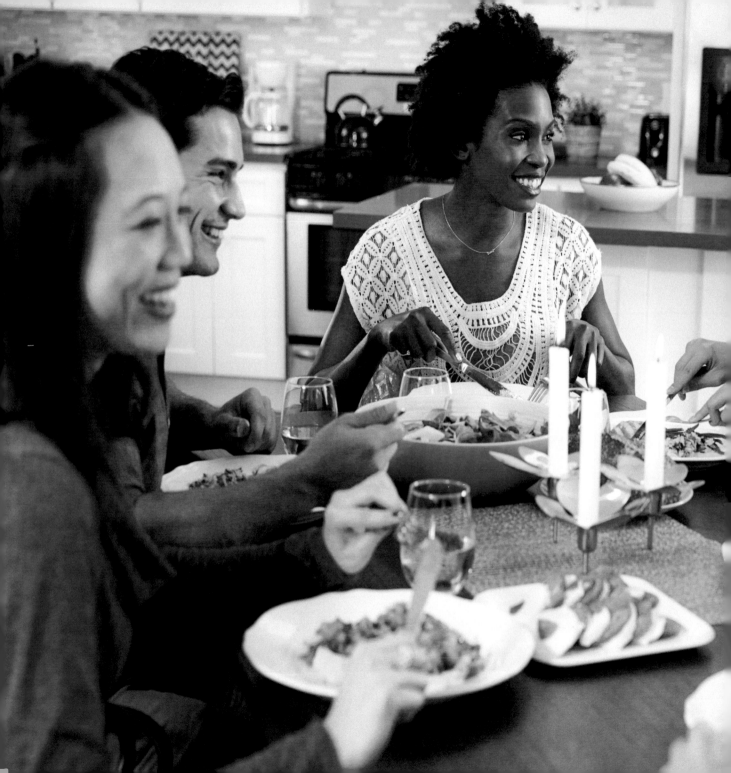

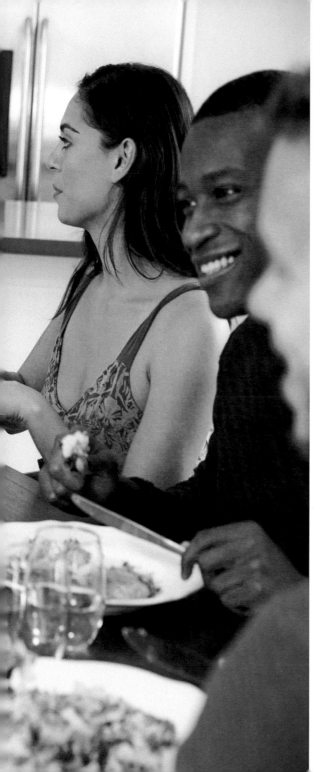

Main &
Side Dishes

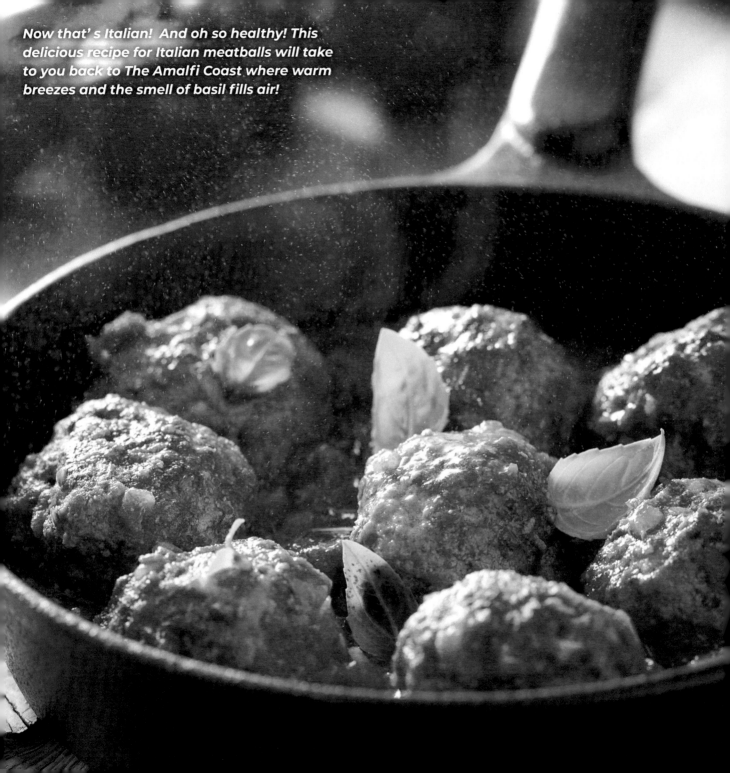

Now that's Italian! And oh so healthy! This delicious recipe for Italian meatballs will take to you back to The Amalfi Coast where warm breezes and the smell of basil fills air!

Smart Italian Meatballs

Ingredients:

2 lb grass-fed ground beef
2 cloves garlic, minced
2 eggs
1 cup grated romano cheese
1.5 tbsp chopped parsley
2 tbs cream cheese

Salt and pepper to taste
2 cups toasted, crumbled, Smartbuns®
1.5 cups lukewarm water
1 cup olive oil
Fresh basil to garnish

Preparation:

1. Combine beef, garlic, eggs, cheese, parsley, salt and pepper in a large bowl.

2. Blend Smartbun® crumbs into meat mixture.

3. Slowly add the water 1/2 cup at a time. The mixture should be very moist but still hold its shape if rolled into meatballs.

4. Shape into meatballs.

5. Heat olive oil in a large skillet.

6. Fry meatballs in batches. When the meatball is very brown and slightly crisp remove from the heat and drain on a paper towel. (If your mixture is too wet, cover the meatballs while they are cooking so that they hold their shape better.)

7. Add to your favorite sauce, top with fresh basil and serve on a Smartbun® for a high protein and high fiber HEALTHY, low carb comfort food

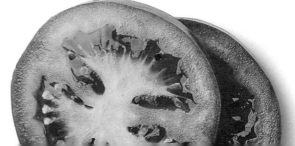

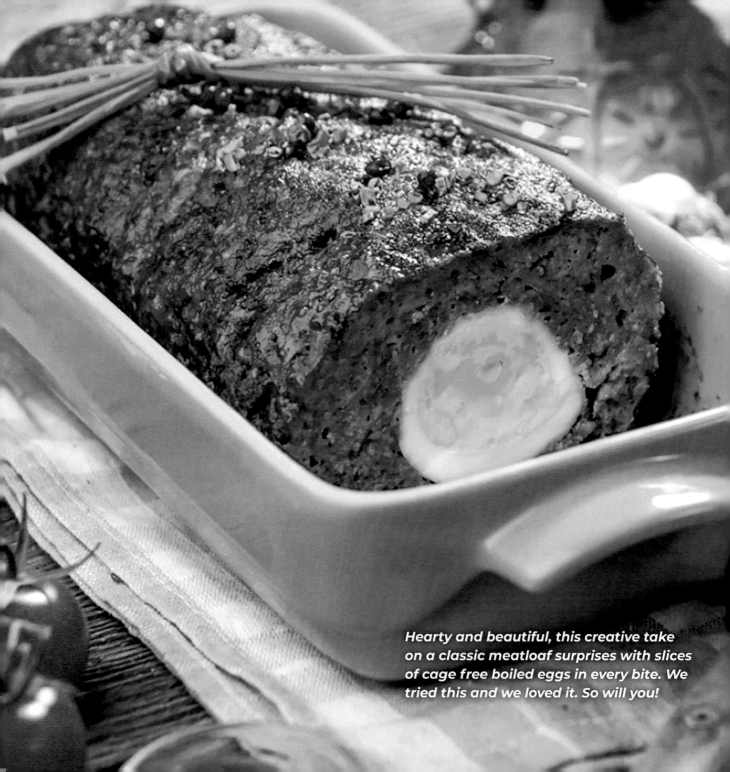

Hearty and beautiful, this creative take on a classic meatloaf surprises with slices of cage free boiled eggs in every bite. We tried this and we loved it. So will you!

Smart Meatloaf

Ingredients:

4 lb lean grass-fed ground beef
4 raw eggs
1 cup crumbled Smartbuns® (plain or sesame for some seeds inside)

3 tsp salt
1 tsp black pepper
2-4 hard-boiled eggs (depending on how much egg you like in each bite)

Preparation:

1. In a large bowl add all the ingredients except the hard-boiled eggs.

2. Mix thoroughly with your hands.

3. Divide the meat mixture into 8 sections. Pat two sections each into a pan (approx. 8' x 4").

4. Lay 2 peeled hard-boiled eggs lengthwise on each of two of the meat rectangles (or one each in the center as a surprise).

5. Cover with remaining meat rectangles and seal edges by pressing together.

6. Gently form the 'meatloaf' into a 'meatloaf' shape with your hands.

7. Roast in a preheated 375 F oven for about 1 1/2 hours or until a meat thermometer reads an internal temp. of 165 F.

8. Let the loaves stand at room temperature about 15 min. before slicing.

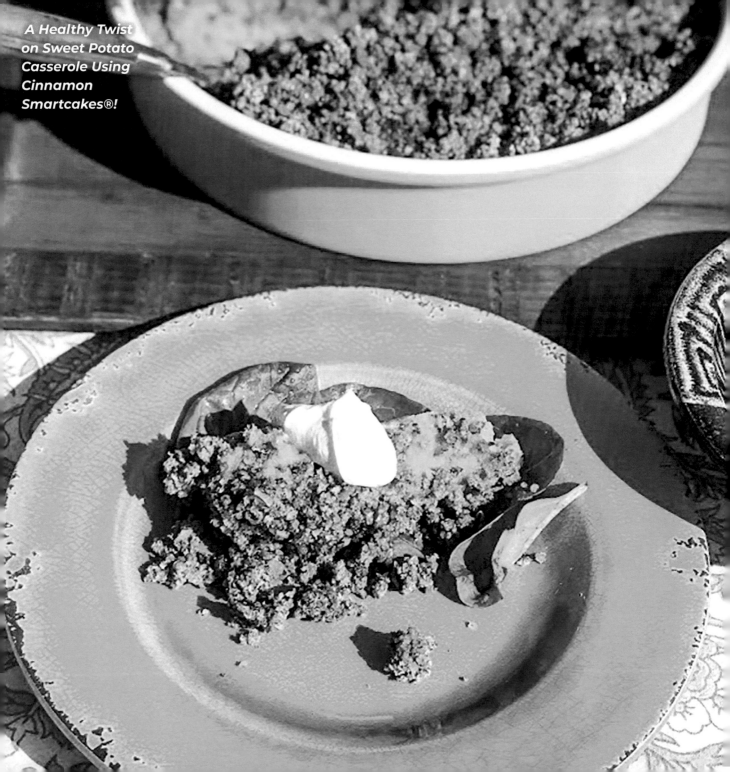

A Healthy Twist on Sweet Potato Casserole Using Cinnamon Smartcakes®!

Jo's Sweet Potato Casserole

Ingredients:

2½ lbs sweet potatoes,
(3 medium - peeled and cut into 2-inch chunks)
2 large eggs
1 tablespoon olive oil
1 tablespoon honey or other/preferred sweetener (optional)
½ cup low-fat milk

2 teaspoons freshly grated orange zest
1 teaspoon vanilla extract
½ teaspoon salt
4 Cinnamon Smartcakes®
½ cup chopped pecans (spices see below)

Preparation:

1. Season the chopped pecans to taste. We used ground nutmeg, cardamon, cloves, and cinnamon. All spice or pumpkin pie spices may be used as a substitute.

2. Place sweet potatoes in a large saucepan and cover with water. Bring to a boil. Cover and cook over medium heat until tender, 10 to 15 minutes. Drain well and return to the pan. Mash with a potato masher.

3. Preheat oven to 350°F.

4. Coat an 8-inch-square (or similar) baking dish with cooking spray.

5. Whisk eggs, oil and honey in a medium bowl. Add mashed sweet potato and mix well. Stir in milk, orange zest, vanilla and salt. Spread the mixture in the prepared baking dish.

6. To prepare topping: Mix crumbled Smartcakes® and crushed pecans (we used a food processor), then sprinkle over the top of the casserole.

7. Bake the casserole until heated through and the top is lightly browned, 10 to 15 minutes.

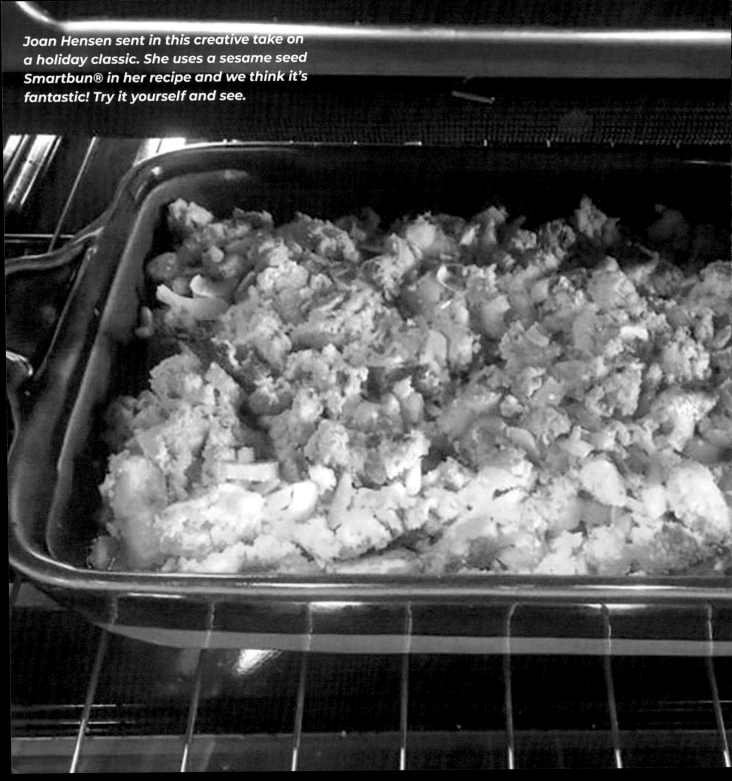

Joan Hensen sent in this creative take on a holiday classic. She uses a sesame seed Smartbun® in her recipe and we think it's fantastic! Try it yourself and see.

Joan's Stunning Stuffing

Ingredients:

4 Smartbuns®, crumbled
4 tbsp butter
2 cups celery, chopped
1 medium onion, chopped

4 cups chicken or vegetable stock
2 tsp salt or chicken/vegetable bouillon
2 tsp dry ground or fresh chopped sage
Salt and pepper to taste

Preparation:

1. Preheat oven to 350 degrees F.

2. Crumble the Smartbuns® in a large bowl.

3. Melt the butter in a large skillet over medium heat.

4. Add the celery and onion and cook until transparent.

5. Mix in the stock, bouillon, and sage and remove from heat.

6. Pour the celery and onion mixture over the crumbled Smartbuns® and mix well. Add salt and pepper to taste.

7. Spread the stuffing into a greased pan and bake until cooked through, about 40 minutes.

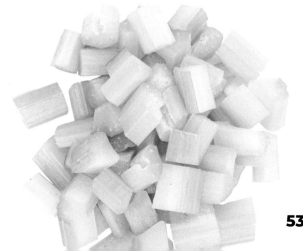

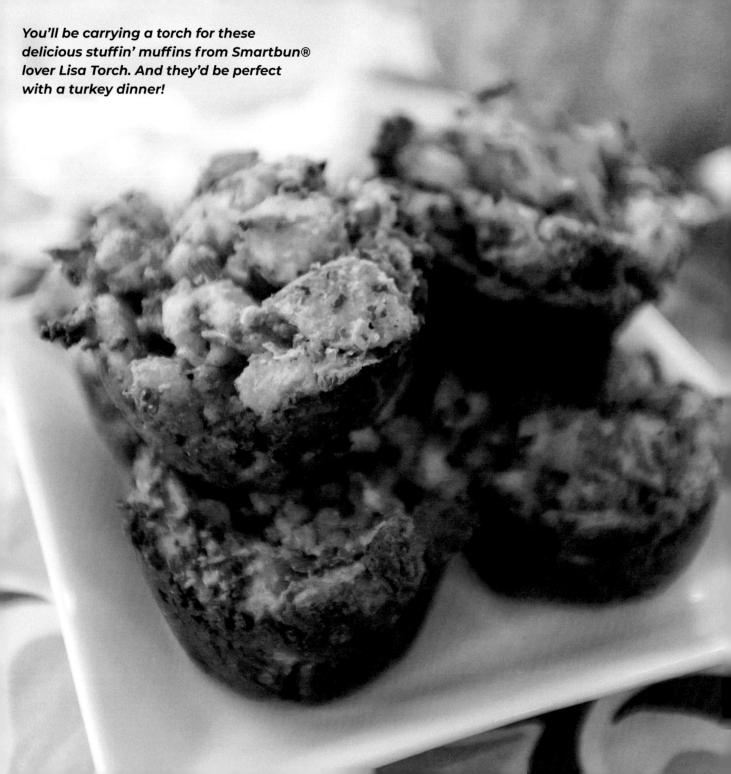

You'll be carrying a torch for these delicious stuffin' muffins from Smartbun® lover Lisa Torch. And they'd be perfect with a turkey dinner!

Lisa's Stuffin' Muffins

Ingredients:

4 large celery sticks - diced
One large onion - finely chopped
Poultry seasoning
Salt & pepper to taste
2 cups chicken or vegetable broth

2 tbsp butter - melted
1/2 cup turkey sausage
8 plain Smartbuns® - cubed
2x6 muffin pan - makes 12 muffins)

Preparation:

1. On medium heat, bring the broth to a boil and let stand on low heat.

2. Melt the butter in a separate skillet or pan and set aside.

3. Preheat oven to 350°F and coat the muffin pan with cooking spray or butter.

4. Sauté the onion and celery in butter until softened.

5. Add turkey sausage and cubed Smartbuns® to a separate pan, mix in the poultry seasoning. Cook on medium heat until turkey sausage is browned.

6. Pour the heated broth and melted butter over the turkey, Smartbun® mixture and incorporate.

7. Continue stirring occasionally until liquid is absorbed.

8. Divide into individual muffin cups and bake at 350°F for 20 minutes or until golden brown. Enjoy!

Photo/Megan M. Dunn

Megan's Bread Pudding

Ingredients:

1 whole egg
1 tbsp heavy cream
1/2 tbsp rosemary - fresh, chopped
1/2 tbsp thyme - fresh, chopped
1/2 tbsp chives - fresh, chopped

1 tbsp parsley - fresh, chopped
1/4 tbsp salt - 1/8 tbsp black pepper
1/8 tbsp granulated garlic
1 link cooked chicken sausage - chopped
1 plain Smartbun® - toasted and cubed

Preparation:

1. In a small mixing bowl, whisk together egg and heavy cream.

2. Crumble the pre-toasted and cubed Smartbun®, fold into it into the egg and cream mixture with the rest of the ingredients.

3. Bake in a small dish at 375°F in the oven for 15-20 minutes.

4. The top will start to brown when it is done, take out and let cool for 10-15 minutes and enjoy!

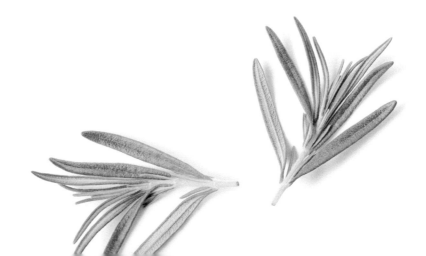

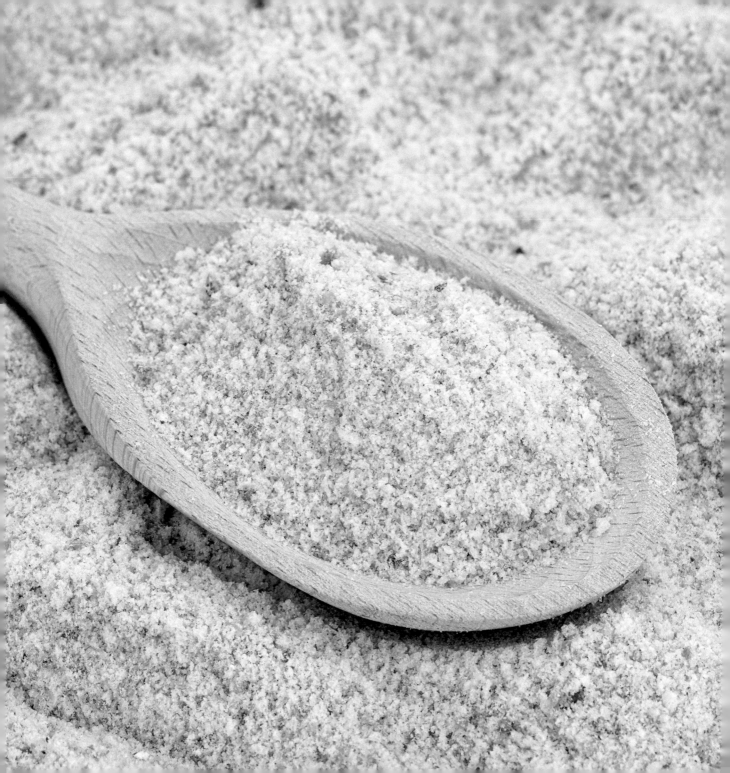

Jo's Stuffed Anything...

Herbed Smartcrumb Stuffing

This base recipe is used to stuff mushroom, clams, oysters, or chicken breast. All these options create great keto friendly appetizers, main dishes, or sides to delight even the most discriminating and non-keto guests!

Ingredients:

2 Tbsp. olive oil
1/2 medium white onion, minced
2 cloves garlic, peeled and minced
1 and ½ cup plain Smartbuns® toasted and chopped fine in a blender or food processor
4 tablespoons unsalted butter, softened
1.2 cup chopped fresh parsley
1 tablespoon finely chopped fresh dill leaves
1 teaspoon finely chopped fresh thyme leaves
1/2 teaspoon finely chopped fresh rosemary leaves
Fresh Ground Pepper

Preparation:

1. Heat olive oil in a saute pan. Cook onion and garlic until translucent, stirring frequently, about 5 minutes. Remove from heat and let cool completely.

2. Stir together onion mixture, Smartbun® breadcrumbs, herbs, and butter in a bowl; season with pepper.

Yield: Makes enough for 16 servings

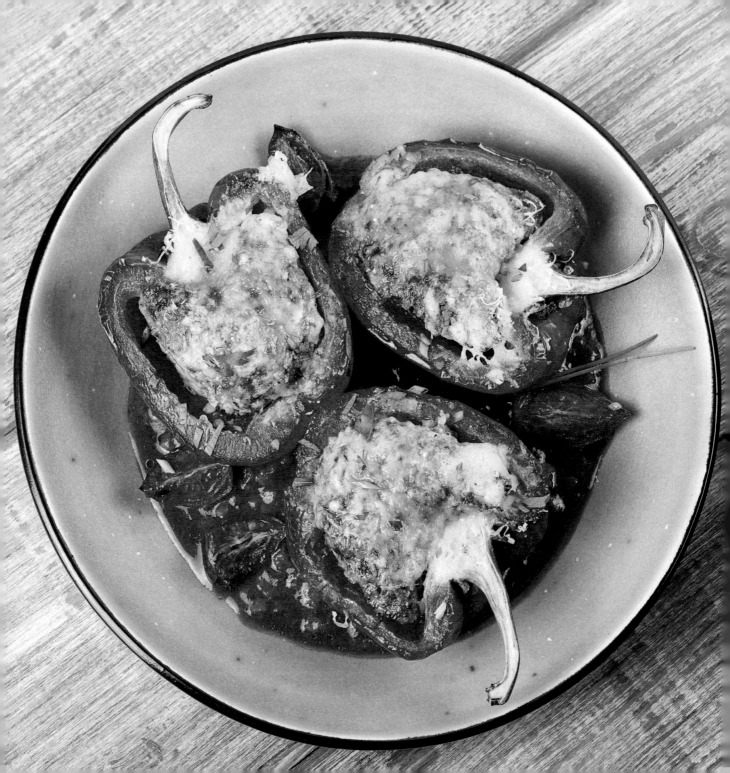

Smart Stuffed Pepper

Ingredients:

1/2 c. Herbed Smartcrumb Stuffing
2 tbsp. extra-virgin olive oil, plus more for drizzling
1 medium onion, chopped
2 tbsp. tomato paste
3 cloves garlic, minced
1 lb. ground chicken, pork or grass-fed beef
1 (14.5-oz.) can diced tomatoes
1 1/2 tsp. dried oregano
Kosher salt
Freshly ground black pepper
6 bell peppers, tops and cores removed
1 c. feta cheese (or substitute your fa

Preparation:

1. Preheat oven to 400°. In a large skillet over medium heat, heat oil. Cook onion until soft, about 5 minutes. Stir in tomato paste and garlic and cook until fragrant, about 1 minute more. Add ground chicken or beef and cook, breaking up meat with a wooden spoon, until no longer pink, 6 minutes. Drain fat.

2. Return chicken or beef mixture to skillet, then stir in Herbed Smartcrumb Stuffing and diced tomatoes. Season with oregano, salt, and pepper. Let simmer until liquid has reduced slightly, about 5 minutes.

3. Place peppers cut side-up in a 9"-x-13" baking dish and drizzle with oil. Spoon beef mixture into each pepper and top with cheese, then cover baking dish with foil.

4. Bake until peppers are tender, about 35 minutes. Uncover and bake until cheese is bubbly, 10 minutes more.

5. Garnish with parsley before serving.

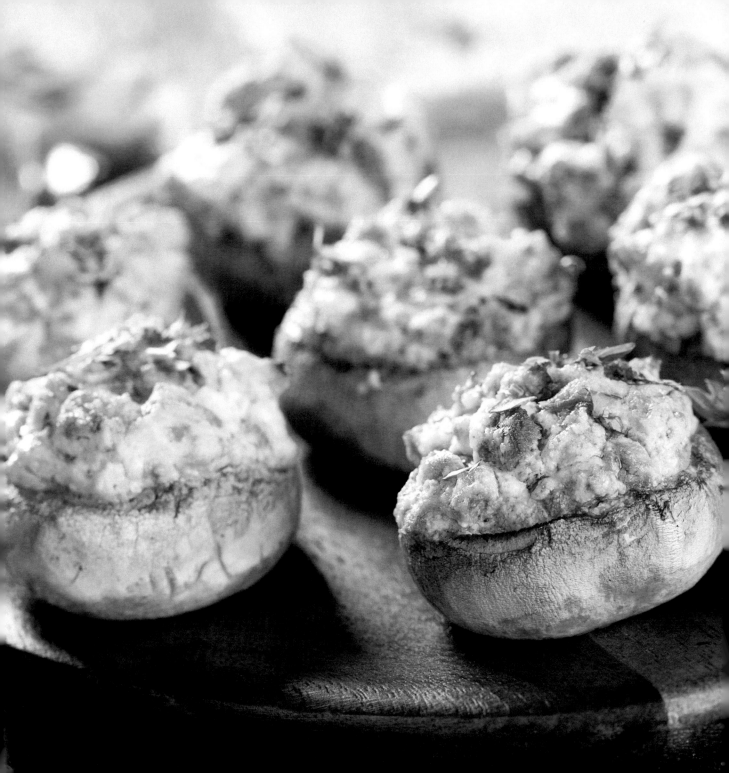

Salmon Stuffed Mushrooms

Salmon is full of omega-3 fatty acids, and mushrooms have vitamin D. Combine them in this appetizer or side dish for a healthy and low-carb treat.

Additional Ingredients:

24 large mushrooms
 2 Tbsp. lemon juice
1 pouch (6 oz.) salmon, drained

Preparation:

1. Preheat oven to 375°F. Clean mushrooms by brushing with a soft brush. Remove the mushroom stems from the caps. Brush the caps with lemon juice and set aside. Trim the ends from the stems and finely chop the stems.

2. In saucepan, heat olive oil over medium heat. Add mushroom stems; cook and stir until tender, about 6 minutes. Remove from heat and place in bowl. Add the Herbed Smartcrumb Stuffing and mix well. Add salmon and mix gently. Stuff this mixture into the mushroom caps.

3. Bake for 25 minutes or until mushrooms are tender and filling is hot and beginning to brown on top. Let cool for 10 minutes, then serve.

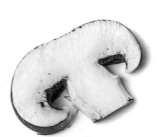
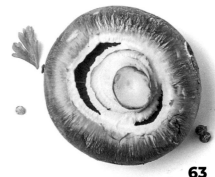

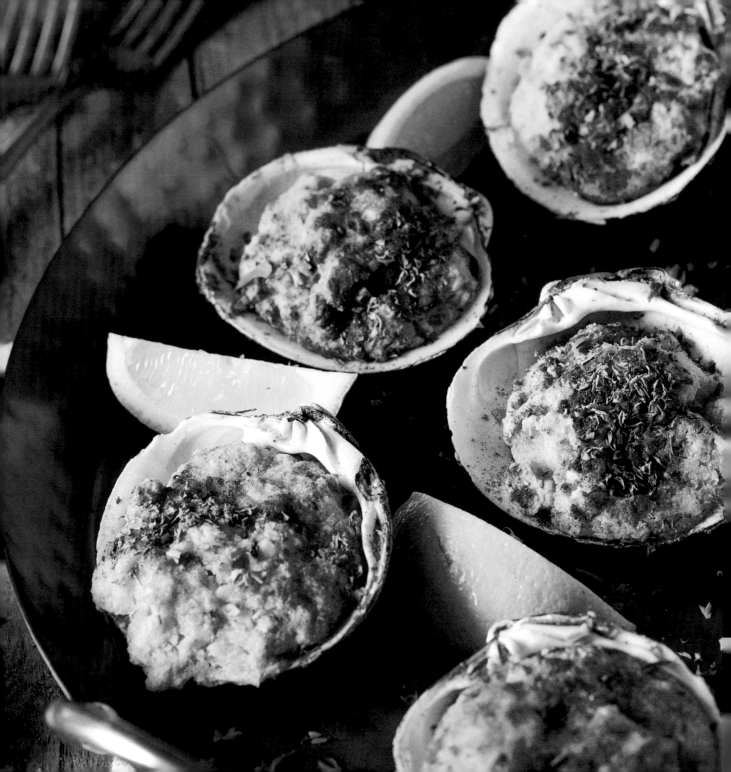

Smart Stuffed Clams

Ingredients:

1 cup Smart Stuffing
16 clams
4 to 6 tablespoons clam broth
(reserved from steaming clams)
 Vegetable or Chicken Stock

Preparation:

1. Heat olive oil in a pot over medium-high heat. Cook onion until softened but not browned, stirring occasionally, about 5 minutes. Add garlic and sauté, stirring, just until fragrant, about 1 minute.

2. Add chicken or vegetable stock and bring to a simmer.

3. Add clams and stir to combine. Cover and steam until clams have opened, 5 to 7 minutes.

4. Remove from heat. Use a slotted spoon to transfer clams to a rimmed baking sheet to cool, discarding any that do not open. Strain clam broth through a fine sieve, and reserve broth for making stuffing.

5. When clams are cool enough to handle, remove all meat, and reserve. Remove half of each clam shell, and discard. Arrange the remaining halves on a rimmed baking sheet. Cut each clam into Â½-inch pieces; return pieces to shell. (Clams can be prepared to this point up to 1 day ahead. Cover with plastic wrap and refrigerate.)

6. Stir into your Herbed Smartcrumb Stuffing just enough clam broth to moisten stuffing.

7. Preheat oven to 350 degrees F. Dividing evenly, press Herbed Breadcrumb Stuffing into clam shells, smoothing with the back of a spoon. Bake until tops are golden, 25 to 30 minutes.

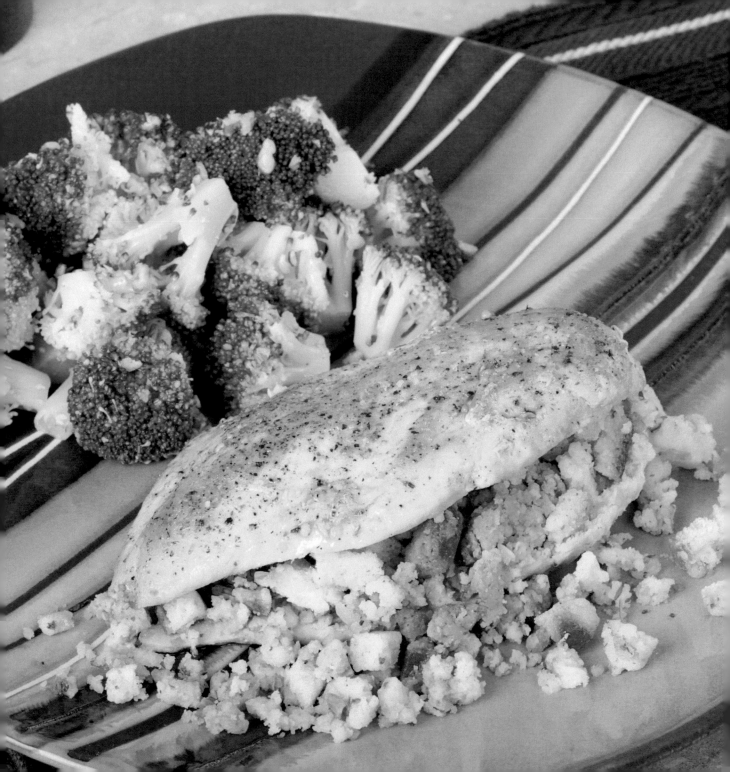

Keto Stuffed Chicken

Ingredients:

1 cup Smart Stuffing
(optionally just chopped instead of blended)
4 chicken breasts
2 tablespoons olive oil

1 Package Frozen Creamed Spinach
(or your own prepared with sour cream, parmesan and spinach)
Salt, Pepper or your favorite seasoning

Preparation:

1. Heat the frozen creamed spinach and mix with the Smart Stuffing.

2. Stuff each breast with up to ¼th of a cup of the spinach dip mixture and then secure the sides of the chicken with wooden toothpicks then season with salt and pepper or your favorite seasoning.

3. Brown the chicken on for 6 minutes per side in a hot skillet with olive oil, and then bake in a hot oven at 375F for 20- 25 minutes or until juice of chicken is clear when center of thickest part is cut (at least 165°F). Remove toothpicks before serving.

4. If you add a vegetable side, sprinkle some of the smart stuffing over it before you bake.

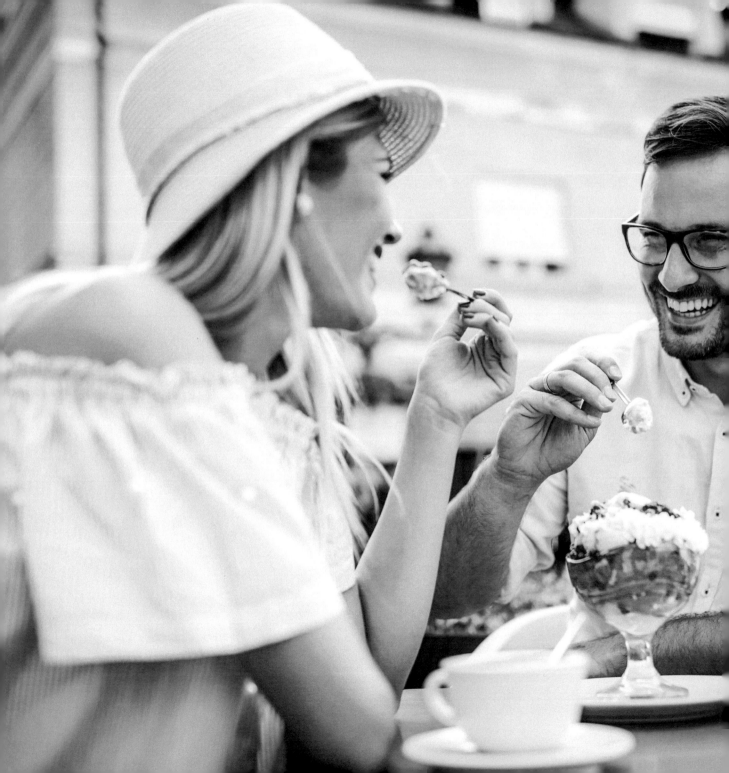

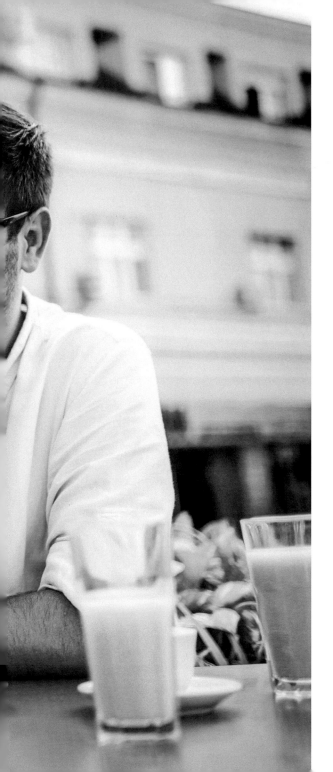

Desserts

Don't trifle with this Trifle! An absolutely delicious AND beautiful dessert presentation from Joanne Walter. We tried this and we LOVED it!

Photo/Joanne Walter

Jo's Tasty Trifle

Ingredients:

3-4* Pumpkin SmartMuf'ns™
3-4 Banana Nut Smartmuf'ns™
2 pints heavy whipping cream
4 cups raw cranberries

orange extract
vanilla extract
monk fruit sweetener (optional)

Preparation:

1. Crumble 3-4 Pumpkin SmartMuf'ns in the base of your Trifle dish. (4 if serving 12 people)

2. Add a layer of cooked, cooled cranberries (about 2 cups)

3. In a blender (or mixer) mix 1 cup of cooked cranberries (cooled) with 1 pint of heavy whipping cream.

4. Layer the pink cream over the Pumpkin SmartMuf'ns.

5. Add 3-4 crumbled Banana Nut SmartMuf'ns. (4 if serving 12 people)

6. Layer the remaining cooled cooked cranberries over the Muf'ns.

7. Rinse your blender and blend the second pint of heavy whipping cream with a dash of vanilla extract.

8. Top of your Trifle dish with the Vanilla Whipped Cream.

9. Let sit in a cool place and serve.

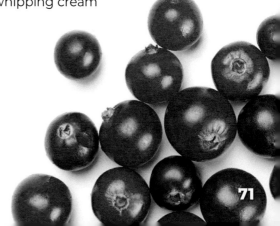

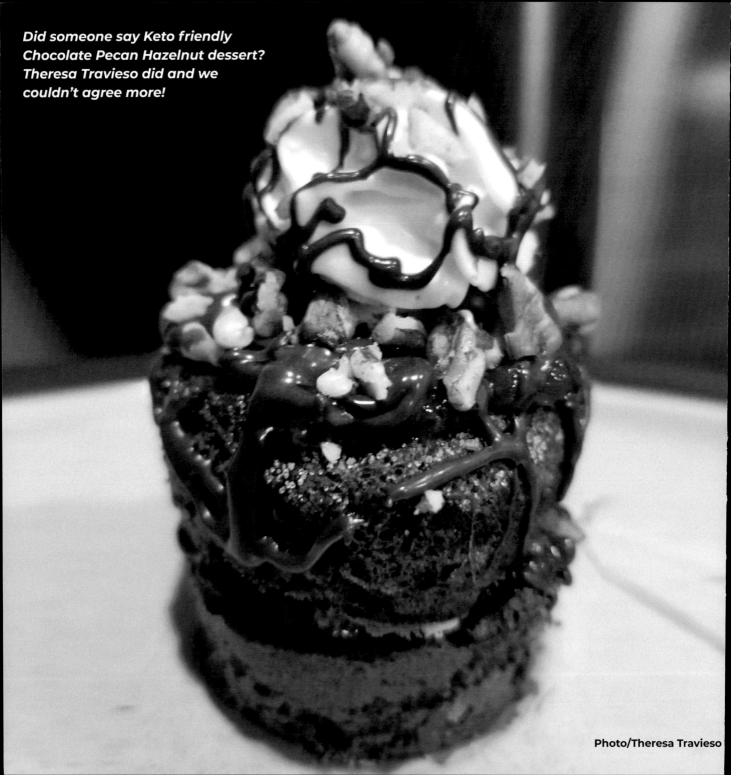

Did someone say Keto friendly Chocolate Pecan Hazelnut dessert? Theresa Travieso did and we couldn't agree more!

Photo/Theresa Travieso

Theresa's Keto Confection

Ingredients:

2 tsp of sugar-free hazelnut spread
2 tsp of chopped pecans
Dairy-free whipped cream
1 two-pack of chocolate Smartcakes®

Preparation:

1. Start by removing the Smartcakes® from their paper wrappers and cut in half horizontally.

2. Heat 2 teaspoons of the sugar-free hazelnut spread in a microwave for approximately 30 seconds or until soft.

3. Place the bottom half of the Smartcake® on your plate or bowl and spread about 1 tsp of the sugar-free hazelnut spread and chopped pecans in middle section.

4. Place the top half of the Smartcake® and repeat. With a spoon, drizzle remaining hazelnut spread and sprinkle remaining chopped pecans.

5. Add a spray of dairy-free whipped cream topping and enjoy!

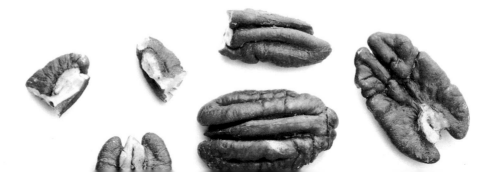

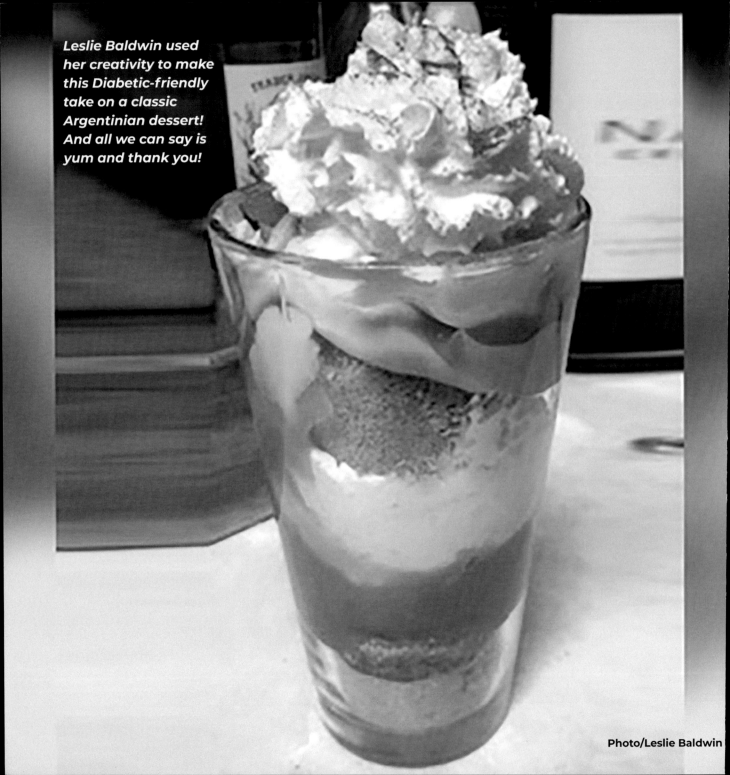

Leslie Baldwin used her creativity to make this Diabetic-friendly take on a classic Argentinian dessert! And all we can say is yum and thank you!

Lesle's Dulce De Leche

Ingredients:

2 Sugar-free Jell-O® Dulce Le Leche pudding cups
Fat-free whipped cream
A pinch of cinnamon spice
2 cinnamon Smartcakes®

Preparation:

1. Remove the Smartcakes® from their paper wrappers and in a clean 32oz 'beer' glass or mason jar place one Cinnamon Smartcake® on the bottom of the glass. Pack it to the bottom lightly.

2. Scoop one Sugar Free Jell-O® Dulce De Leche Pudding Cup on top of the Smartcake®.

3. Cover with Fat Free Whipped Cream and repeat for the top layers.

4. Enjoy your dessert and remember that you're NOT cheating!!!

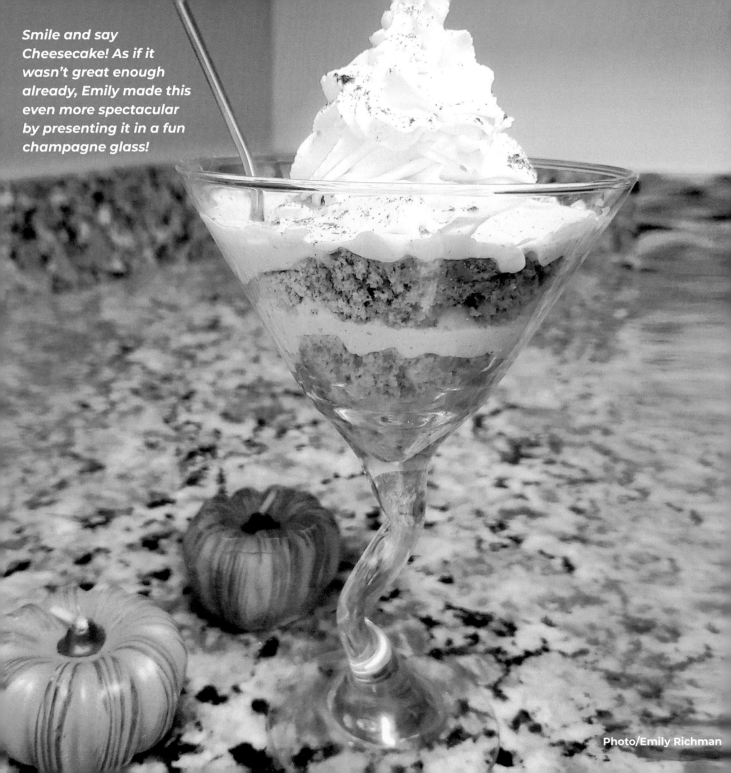

Smile and say Cheesecake! As if it wasn't great enough already, Emily made this even more spectacular by presenting it in a fun champagne glass!

Photo/Emily Richman

Emily's Cheesecake Parfait

Ingredients:

2 oz cream cheese
6 tbsp whipped cream
60g pumpkin puree

1.5 tbsp monkfruit sweetener
1/2 tsp pumpkin pie spice
1 cinnamon Smartcake®

Preparation:

1. Using a mixer and large bowl, whip the 4 tbsp of whipped cream, cream cheese, pumpkin puree, monk fruit, and pumpkin pie spice until blended smooth and creamy.

2. Then remove the Smartcakes® from their paper wrappers and cut in half horizontally.

3. Crumble lower half of Cinnamon Smartcake® at the bottom of a martini glass or dessert dish.

4. Spoon or pipe half of the pumpkin mixture on top.

5. Repeat step with the remaining top half of the Cinnamon Smartcake® and pumpkin mixture.

6. Top with 2 tbsp of whipped cream and sprinkle pumpkin pie spice on top for garnish - enjoy!

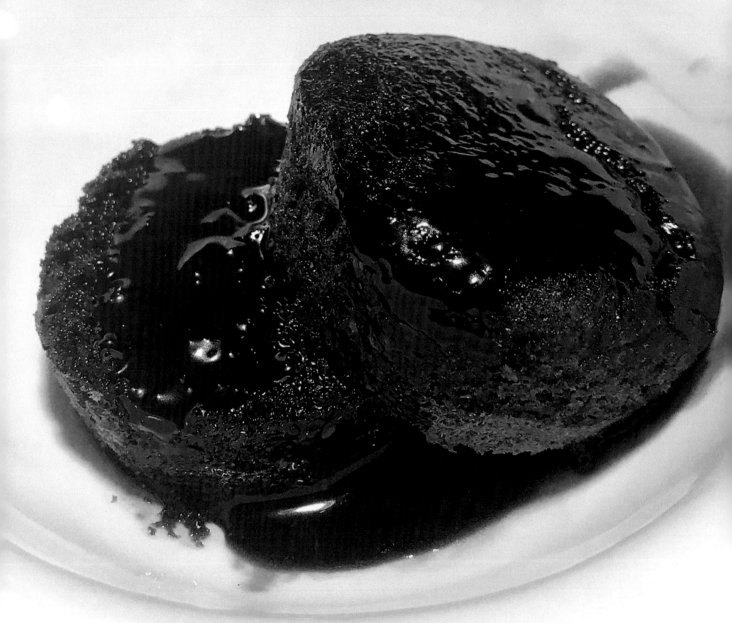

Rachel Collins offered up this wonderful treat that she calls Easy Keto Chocolate Fudge Smartcakes®. We just call it delicious!

Photo/Mellanie DeLeon

Rachel's Chocolate Fudge

Ingredients:

2 tbsp of sugar-free chocolate syrup
1 two-pack of chocolate Smartcakes®
(Optional toppings: sugar-free whipped cream, sugar-free sprinkles.)

Preparation:

1. Start by removing the Smartcakes® from their paper wrappers and cut in half horizontally.

2. Place the Smartcakes® in the microwave and heat for approximately 15-20 seconds.

3. Place the lower half of the Smartcake® into the bottom layer of your cup or container.

4. Top with sugar-free syrup and any other desired toppings.

5. Repeat for the other half, top it off with sugar-free whipped cream, and enjoy!

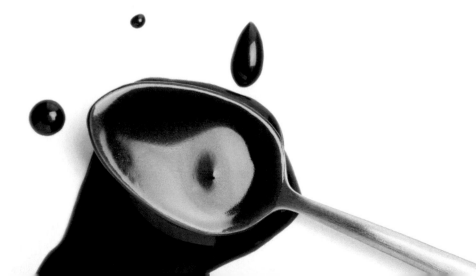

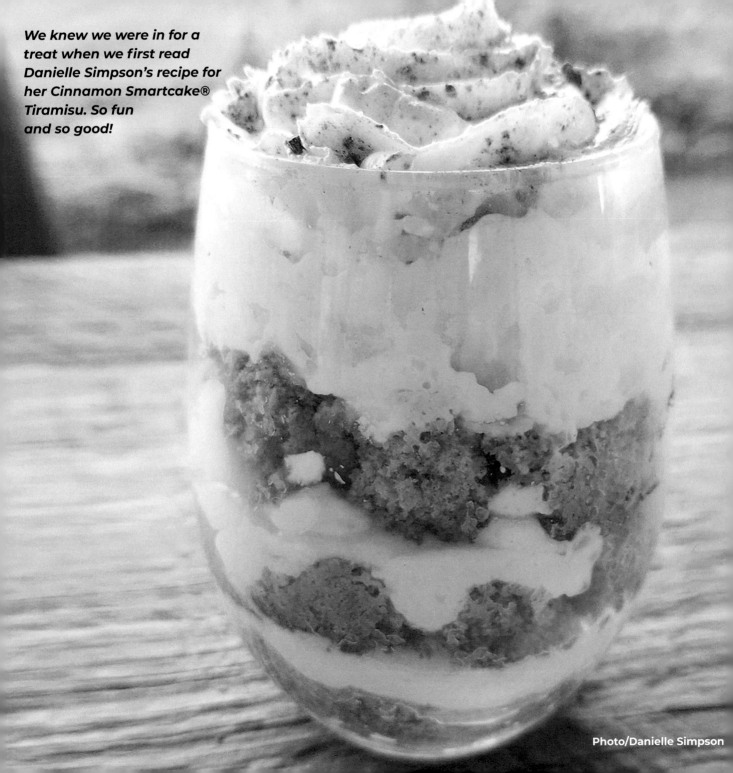

We knew we were in for a treat when we first read Danielle Simpson's recipe for her Cinnamon Smartcake® Tiramisu. So fun and so good!

Photo/Danielle Simpson

Danielle's Tiramisu

Ingredients:

1 cup whipped cream
3⁄4 cup mascarpone
13⁄4 cup heavy whipping cream
Espresso drizzle

3⁄4 cup espresso
3 tbsp sweetener (optional)
A pinch of cocoa powder topping
6 cinnamon Smartcakes®

Preparation:

1. Preheat oven to 350°F.

2. Then remove the Smartcakes® from their paper wrappers and cut into squares (your choice size, we went with smaller pieces so they would have a drier texture).

3. Place Smartcake® slices on a baking sheet and bake for 15-20 minutes or until they're dried out (the texture should not be crumbly or falling apart).

4. In a large mixing bowl, mix mascarpone or cream cheese with heavy whipping cream until firm and add sweetener to taste.

5. Layer Smartcake® squares on the bottom of an individual serving glass, drizzle with the espresso.

6. Top with the filling.

7. Sprinkle with cocoa powder, or grated chocolate

8. Repeat the above steps for 2-3 layers.

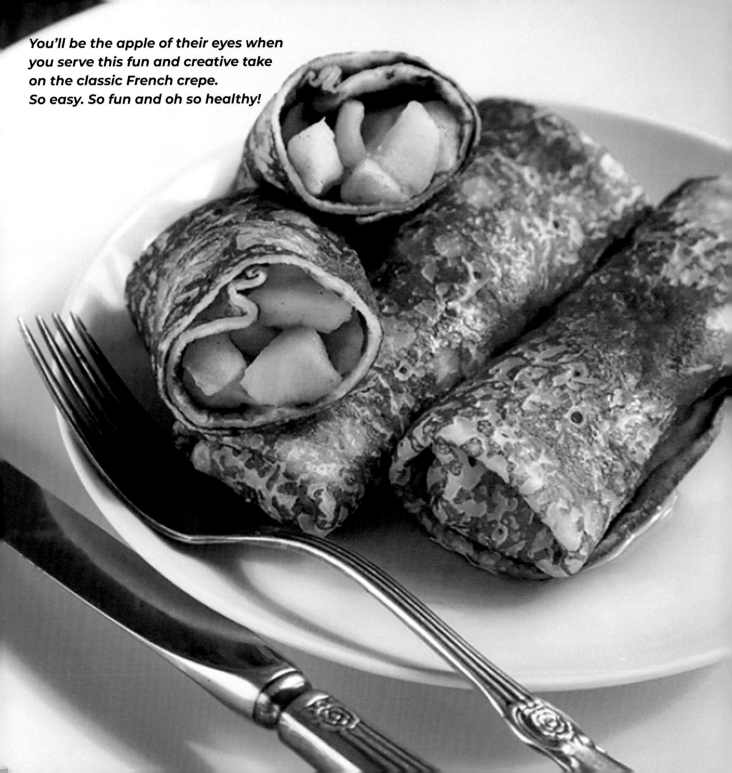

You'll be the apple of their eyes when you serve this fun and creative take on the classic French crepe.
So easy. So fun and oh so healthy!

Smart Apple Crepes

Ingredients:

2 eggs
2 oz cream cheese
1 cinnamon Smartcake®
1 cooked apple (for the filling)

Preparation:

1. Combine 2 eggs, 2 ounces of cream cheese and one Cinnamon Smartcake® per serving. This high protein, low carb treat lets you enjoy and decadent treat without the carbs to bog your system down or the glutens.

2. Combine the eggs, cream cheese and Smartcake® in a strong blender or mixer. and pour the batter in a lightly oiled and heated crepe or frying pan (low heat). Coconut oil works well. Tilt the pan with a circular motion so that the batter coats the surface evenly.

3. Fry over medium high heat for about 2 minutes, until the bottom is light brown. Loosen with a spatula, turn and cook the other side.

4. Filling: Peel 2 apples and dice. Sprinkle with cinnamon. Heat them in a saute pan coated with coconut oil and a 3 tablespoons of water for 6-7 minutes or less if you want a firmer filling.

5. Wrap the apple filling in the crepes and serve!

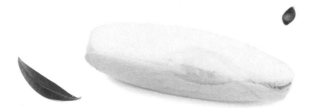

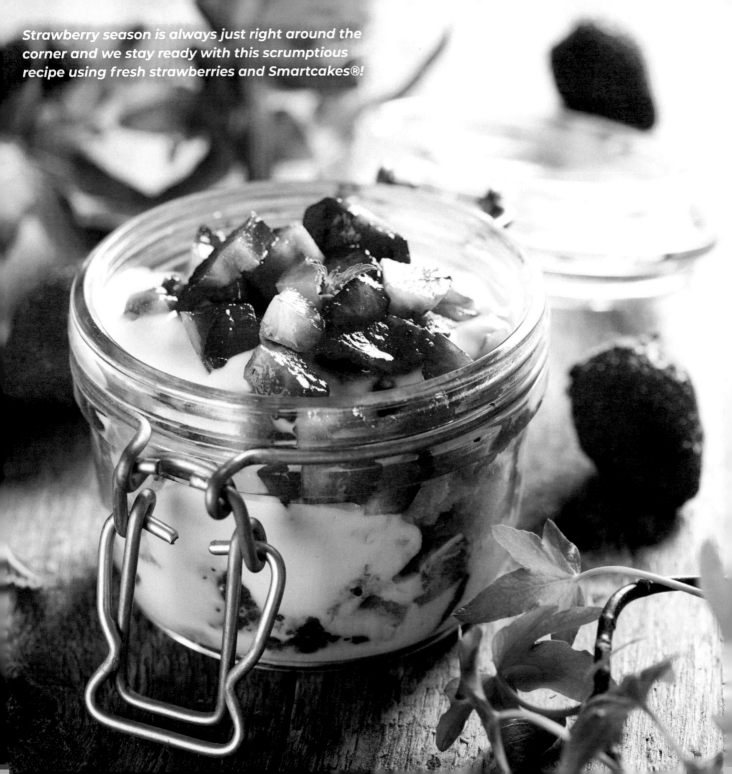

Strawberry season is always just right around the corner and we stay ready with this scrumptious recipe using fresh strawberries and Smartcakes®!

Smart Strawberry Trifle

Ingredients:

1 chocolate Smartcake®
1 raspberry Smartcake®
4 tbsp unsweetened whipped heavy cream. Add stevia to taste (optional)
1 cup fresh strawberries, sliced dash cocoa powder

Preparation:

1. Heat strawberries over low heat until a sauce is formed. Stir frequently.

2. Scoop two, full tbsp. of the fresh, strawberry sauce into the Mason jar as the first layer.

3. Take the Chocolate Smartcake® out of its cup and gently press into the mason jar as the second layer, breaking it a little, so the cake has the chance to soak up the strawberry sauce.

4. Add 2 tbsp. of heavy whipping cream then arrange some of the strawberry slices on top and repeat all the steps starting with the strawberry sauce, but this time adding the Raspberry Smartcake®.

5. Finish off with one final tbsp. of heavy whipping cream and dust of cocoa powder and slice of strawberry.

6. Refrigerate for an hour and serve.

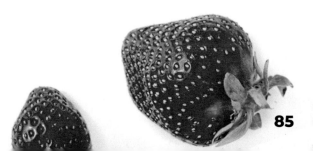

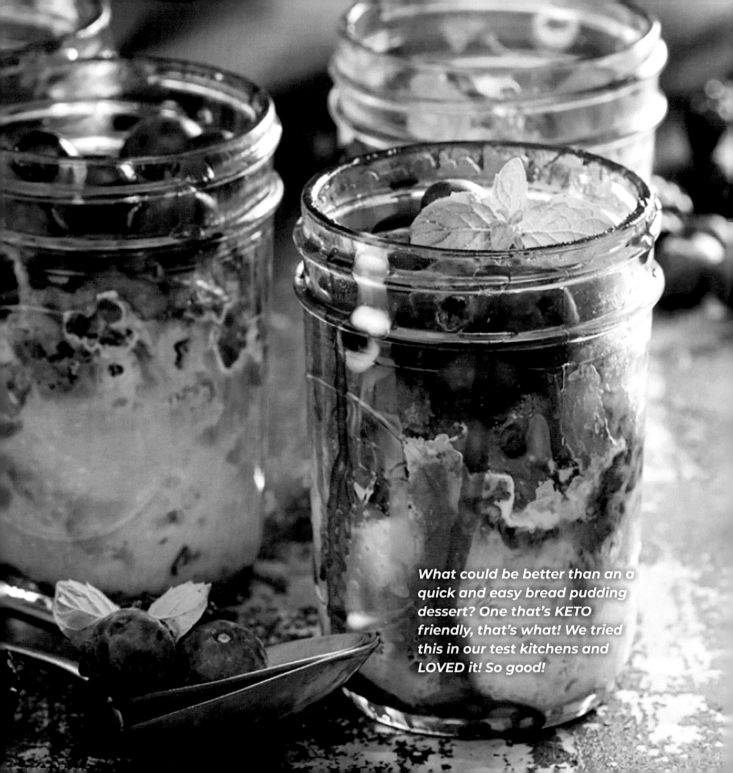

What could be better than an a quick and easy bread pudding dessert? One that's KETO friendly, that's what! We tried this in our test kitchens and LOVED it! So good!

Smart Bread Pudding

Ingredients:

Pudding
1 cup cinnamon Smartcakes®
1.5 cups unsweetened coconut milk
1.5 cups unsweetened apple sauce
2 whole eggs, lightly beaten
1 red delicious apple, peel on, diced
1/4 cup walnuts

Sauce
3 Scoops vanilla whey protein powder
1/4 cup fat-free plain yogurt
1/4 cup coconut milk
1/4 cup blueberries (garnish)

Preparation:

1. In a large mixing bowl, add coconut milk, unsweetened applesauce and eggs. Whisk.

2. Fold in Smartbun® cubes, walnuts, and apples.

3. Transfer to oven safe dish, cover and refrigerate one hour.

4. Preheat oven to 350F and bake until it's set and the top turns golden brown (about 45 minutes). Remove and cool to room temperature.

5. Transfer to mason jars and refrigerator.

6. Make the sauce by adding protein powder and yogurt to a mixing bowl and mix until incorporated.

7. Add milk and stir until creamy.

8. Pour generously over bread pudding.

9. Add fresh blueberries and a sprig of mint to garnish.

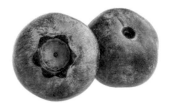

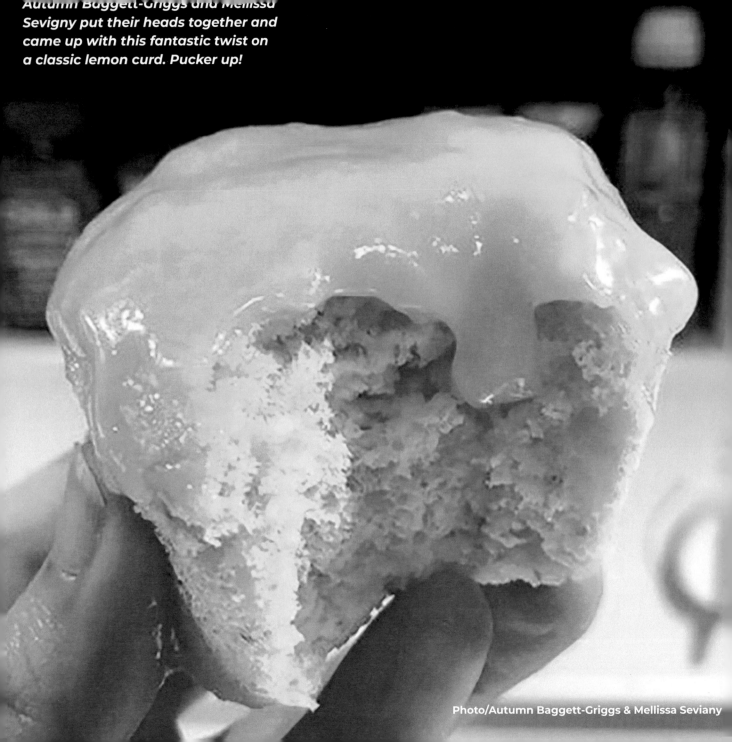

Autumn Baggett-Griggs and Mellissa Sevigny put their heads together and came up with this fantastic twist on a classic lemon curd. Pucker up!

Photo/Autumn Baggett-Griggs & Mellissa Seviany

Two Girls Lemon Curd

Ingredients:

1/2 stick butter
1/4 cup of sugar-free sweetener
1/4 cup fresh lemon juice

1/8 cup lemon zest
3 egg yolks
1 two-pack of lemon Smartcakes®

Preparation:

1. Melt the butter in a saucepan on low heat.

2. Once melted, remove from heat and whisk in the sweetener little by little.

3. Add lemon juice and lemon zest until dissolved and then whisk in egg yolks.

4. Return to stove over low heat. Continue whisking while cooking, until the curd mixture thickens. (It's very important to keep the ingredients moving, so they don't cook into solid clumps!)

5. Remove from heat and let cool to room temperature. Once cooled, cover and store in the fridge for up to one month.(But we can guarantee it will not
last an entire week, if you love lemon curd like we do!)

6. Top your Smartcake® with the lemon curd! We have selected the Lemon Smartcakes® for this recipe, but this will work well with any of our flavors! (Optional: Top with sugar free whipped cream and berries and serve with tea or sparkling water.)

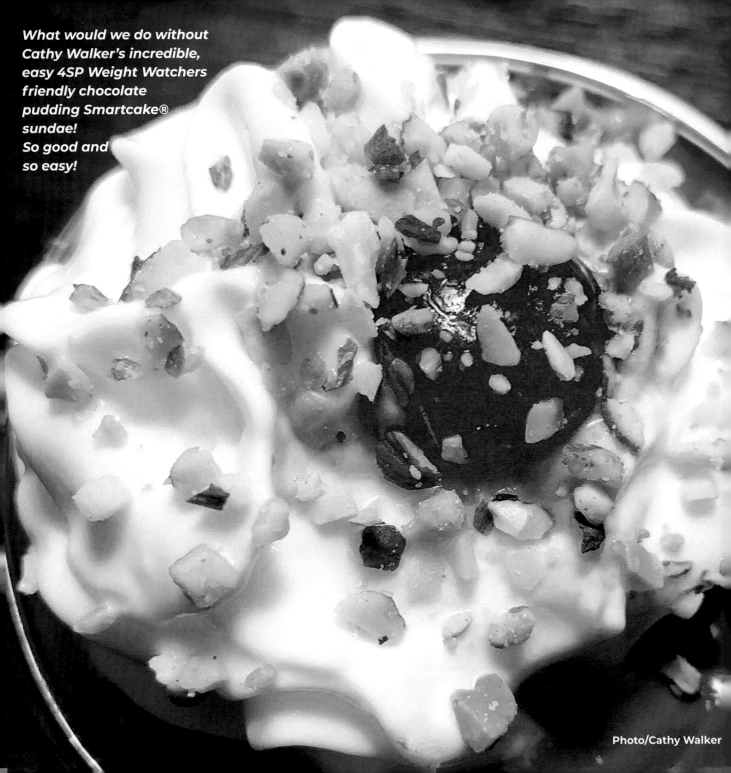

What would we do without Cathy Walker's incredible, easy 4SP Weight Watchers friendly chocolate pudding Smartcake® sundae! So good and so easy!

Photo/Cathy Walker

Cathy's Chocolate Sundae

Ingredients:

1 cup sugar-free, Jell-O® Chocolate Pudding
1 two-pack of Smartcakes® flavor of your choosing
½ cup of chopped peanuts, walnuts, or pecans
(optional toppings: sugar-free whipped cream and your favorite cherry on top!)

Preparation:

1. Start by removing the Smartcakes® from their paper wrappers and heat in the microwave for approximately 10 seconds.

2. Spoon on your choice of instant sugar-free chocolate pudding on top of the Smartcakes®.

3. Spoon or pipe on the sugar-free whipped cream.

4. Sprinkle on your choice of unsalted and unseasoned chopped nuts.

5. Top it all off with a cherry and enjoy!

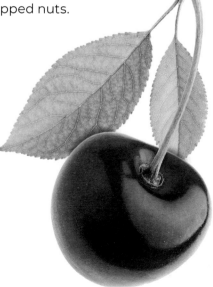

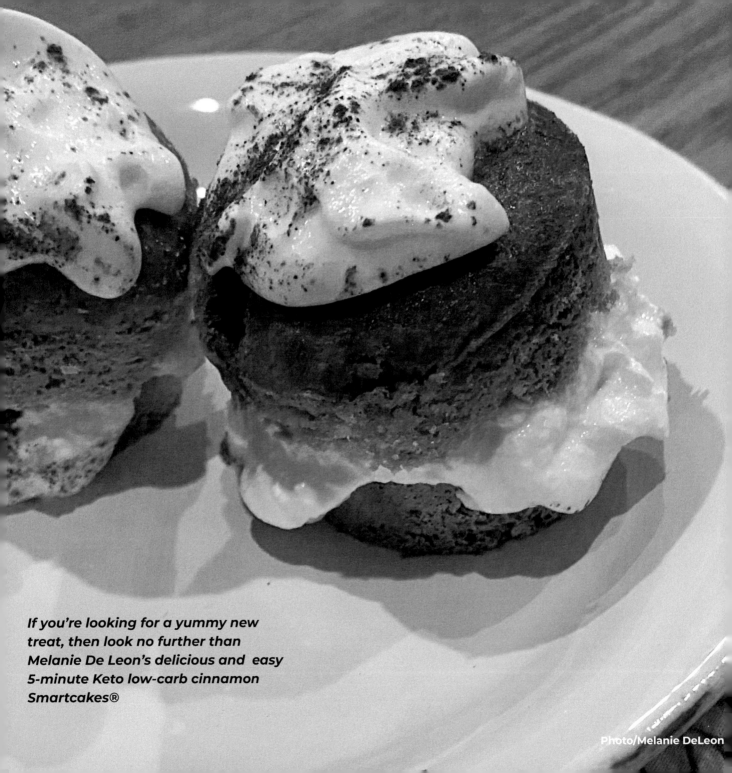

If you're looking for a yummy new treat, then look no further than Melanie De Leon's delicious and easy 5-minute Keto low-carb cinnamon Smartcakes®

Photo/Melanie DeLeon

Melanie's Cinnamon Snack

Ingredients:

4 oz of cream cheese - softened
1/2 cup sugar-free powdered sugar
1 tsp of vanilla extract

4 oz of cream cheese - softened
1/2 cup sugar-free powdered sugar
1 tsp of vanilla extract

Preparation:

1. Mix butter and cream cheese. The mixture should be overall smooth with no clumps.

2. Whisk in the heavy whipping cream and vanilla. (Feel free to add more heavy whipping cream for desired consistency or taste.)

3. Dress up your Smartcakes® with these and enjoy!

4. Try Mellanie's yummy topping on any flavor of Smartcake®! We've tried it on all 5 and they're all amazing!

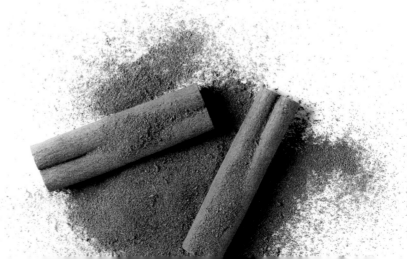

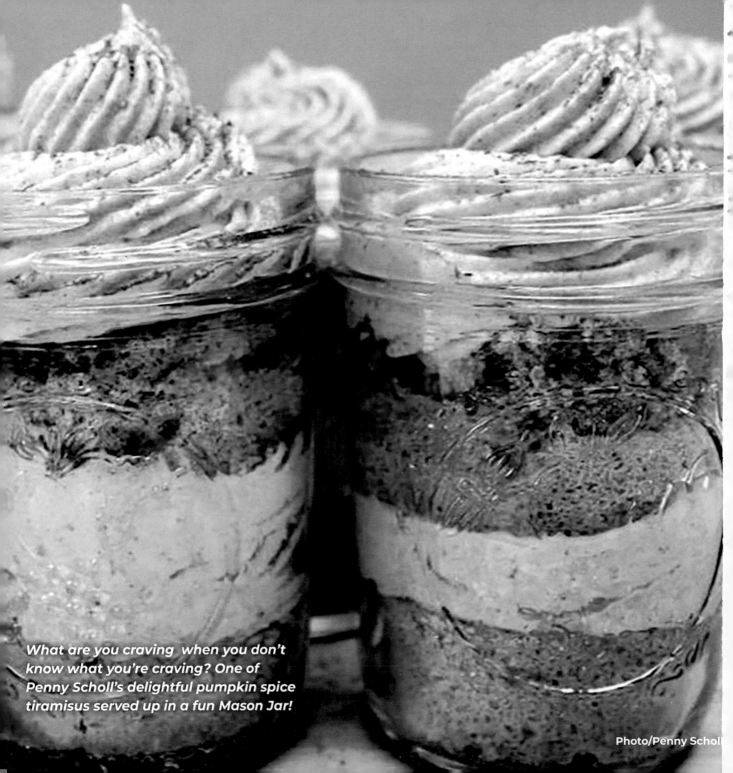

What are you craving when you don't know what you're craving? One of Penny Scholl's delightful pumpkin spice tiramisus served up in a fun Mason Jar!